"*Heart Disease & Hypertension* is a must-read book for everyone. In this book, author Bryant Lusk does an amazing job of explaining, in the most basic terms, the biology behind coronary heart disease and how it links to hypertension. The simple diagrams and descriptions help the reader to understand how the cardiovascular system works. . . . This book will be an eye-opener to most people who read it. The format of the book is wonderfully done, and Lusk's easy-to-read and comprehend writing is refreshing. . . . I recommend *Heart Disease & Hypertension* to anyone who wants to keep or get themselves or their loved ones heart-healthy. This is a book that can be read by all ages. The more we understand our bodies, the more we can do to keep them healthy."

—**Kristi Elizabeth**, San Francisco Book Review

★ ★ ★ ★ ★

"In his book, *Heart Disease & Hypertension*, Bryant Lusk offers approachable content that anyone can understand. . . . *Heart Disease & Hypertension* is an articulate health guide that contains helpful information for ensuring and maintaining heart health. Its comprehensive content will be useful for patients with heart disease looking for ways to reverse the condition and anyone seeking straightforward information on preventing heart disease."

—**Edith Wairimu**, Readers' Favorite

★ ★ ★ ★ ★

"My mother died from a heart attack at a fairly young age, and as far as any of us knew, she did not have any pre-existing conditions. . . . *Heart Disease & Hypertension* is the book I wish I'd had eight years ago . . . But it is not too late for me, and it is not too late for any reader, even if they are advanced in the deterioration of heart health. Most of the advice is easy to implement, and the inclusion of an actual schedule takes this a step further. I also appreciate that spiritual health is mentioned in an inclusive way, and the clickbait and articles that say vitamins are useless are tackled head-on. I don't know a single reader who would not benefit from Lusk's expertise, and I am grateful to have found this book. Better late than never, right? Very highly recommended."

—**Asher Syed**, Readers' Favorite

★ ★ ★ ★ ★

"Bryant Lusk is keenly aware that people typically will not keep up with a complicated routine. Therefore, in *Heart Disease & Hypertension: Vitamin Therapy for a Healthy Heart*, he offers small steps to achieve a healthy heart. Heart disease is a killer, and Bryant wants to save lives. . . . After making sure the reader understands the problem, Bryant dedicates the rest of the book to answers.

"If you had the choice of taking chemicals or natural substances to take care of your heart, which would you choose? Of course, if you are like most people, you probably will choose natural remedies. That is the course for proper heart care that Bryant Lusk presents in *Heart Disease & Hypertension: Vitamin Therapy for a Healthy Heart*. . . . Bryant writes in language that is easy for the layman to understand. Even when he is being technical, he explains all he writes. As a result, I now have more information at my fingertips concerning vitamins and minerals than I have had in studying them for better health for the past fifteen years."

—**Philip Van Heusen**, Readers' Favorite

★ ★ ★ ★ ★

"Bryant Lusk's *Heart Disease & Hypertension* is an informative medical text that delves into supplemental physiology, organ health, and life longevity. . . . the text is accessible because of its bullet point organization and open tone. . . . It is encouraging, too: it suggests that audiences listen to their bodies and account for their individual needs. The dangers and likelihood of overdosing are pronounced with clarity, as are social stressors around physical health, like Covid-19 and toxic relationships. . . . Throughout, the book encourages taking the 'path of least resistance' to prevent cardiovascular issues. While methods like exercise and healthy eating are mentioned, they are not the book's focus. It is more scientific and detailed in covering information that's crucial to understanding the nuances of heart health. . . . "

—**Aleena Ortiz**, Clarion Review
Clarion Rating: 4 out of 5

"*Heart Disease & Hypertension: Vitamin Therapy for a Healthy Heart* links the topics of vitamin therapy, hypertension, and heart disease. While many consumers may well know that the latter conditions hold entwined connections, adding the option of vitamin therapy to affect both is different. . . . Readers should be prepared to absorb the material with an eye to embarking on a lifetime regimen of vitamin-based therapy to improve not just heart conditions but overall bodily system health.

"The real meat of these discussions lies in specific technical details . . . Footnoted references provide the technical research and statistics backing Lusk's contentions, making *Heart Disease & Hypertension* another important tool in the arsenal of fighting the war against heart disease."

—**Donovan's Bookshelf**

". . . negligence of the heart has resulted in disastrous consequences for unsuspecting victims. However, there is hope. . . . *Heart Disease & Hypertension: Vitamin Therapy for a Healthy Heart* by Bryant Lusk not only explains to you why this happens but also gives knowledge-filled advice on how to mitigate it. His vitamin therapy is based on well-researched scientific facts, and the solutions are practicable and sustainable. I can promise that this book is worth it . . . This book is for readers who value their health (which I believe is everyone), especially those interested in understanding how the heart functions and how what we ingest contributes to our health. Vegetarians and vegans are not left out. Finally, I will rate this book a 4 out of 4. The knowledge within, its simplicity, the absence of errors, and the author's passion to impact lives all make this book a must-read."

—**Online Book Club**

Heart Disease & Hypertension:
Vitamin Therapy for a Healthy Heart
by Bryant Lusk

© Copyright 2022 Bryant Lusk

ISBN 978-1-64663-631-0

Library of Congress Control Number: 2021901429

The views of the author are those of the author alone and not necessarily those of any organization or individual mentioned or cited throughout the entirety of this work.

This publication is not intended as a substitute for the medical advice of health-care professionals. Always consult with a physician regarding health matters and particularly with respect to any symptoms that may require medical attention.

Published by

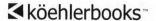

3705 Shore Drive
Virginia Beach, VA 23455
800-435-4811
www.koehlerbooks.com

HEART DISEASE & HYPERTENSION

VITAMIN THERAPY FOR A HEALTHY HEART

BRYANT LUSK

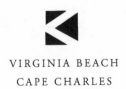

VIRGINIA BEACH
CAPE CHARLES

To Kent and Cheryl. You are my inspiration.

CONTENTS

LIST OF TABLES

LIST OF FIGURES

SINCERE ACKNOWLEDGMENTS

THE FOLLOWING INSTITUTIONS MAINTAIN MUCH of the research used to support this work. Their members work tirelessly behind the scenes to improve the health and well-being of us all.

- Anxiety & Depression Association of America (ADAA)
- Centers for Disease Control and Prevention (CDC)
- Drug-Induced Liver Injury Network (DILIN)
- Food and Drug Administration (FDA)
- National Center for Health Statistics (NCHS)
- National Institutes of Health (NIH)
- National Institute of Mental Health (NIMH)
- National Library of Medicine (NLM)
- Office of Dietary Supplements (ODS)
- World Health Organization (WHO)

Additionally, every medical professional and their staff deserve recognition for their momentous contributions to our health and quality of life. I thank each and every one of you.

No author produces a work they can be truly proud of without significant assistance from others. Special thanks to Ann Bridges, my lead editor, and Cherie Foxley. I appreciate you and everything you've done to help me finish this book.

> "Heart disease is the leading cause of death for men, women, and people of most racial and ethnic groups in the United States.
>
> One person dies every 37 seconds in the United States from cardiovascular disease.
>
> Heart disease costs the United States about $219 billion each year from 2014 to 2015. This includes the cost of health care services, medicines, and lost productivity due to death."
>
> —Centers for Disease Control and Prevention (CDC)

INTRODUCTION

THE HUMAN HEART PUMPS LIFE-GIVING blood every minute of every day for your entire life. Sadly, heart disease is the number one killer of women and men in America and nations abroad. High blood pressure (hypertension) increases the risk.

The terms *heart disease* and *cardiovascular disease* refer to a variety of medical conditions impacting the heart or blood vessels. Some are debilitating, while others can be fatal. Little-known, extremely important facts are revealed in this book to prevent and reverse the most common causes of heart attacks and strokes. You will find simple, readily available options to protect your heart and add years to your life.

Many individuals are not aware of specific vitamin, mineral, and plant-based chemical deficiencies that can cause or contribute to heart disease. Avoiding or reversing these deficiencies can dramatically lower the risk of you and your loved ones succumbing to a heart attack or cardiac arrest. Doing so can also prevent or reverse hypertension and other adverse health conditions.

As a credentialed Safety Inspector and Quality Control Specialist, I examined complex processes to find deficiencies and conflicts within them. As with the bone-building process discussed in my previous book, *Osteoporosis & Osteopenia: Vitamin Therapy for Stronger Bones*, the heart and coronary arteries' biochemical processes are incredible.

The information offered here provides a path of least resistance to a healthier heart and longer life. Moreover, the strategy presented will enable you to achieve long-term results, with only the smallest investments in your health. I am keenly aware of human factors that lead to the failure of overly burdensome routines. My goal is to share an enjoyable and straightforward approach toward significantly improving or maintaining excellent heart function and cardiovascular health.

There are many factors involved in developing hypertension and cardiovascular disease, such as lifestyle and genetics. Chronic deficiencies in organic chemicals, vitamins, and minerals are a significant factor you can easily control. Moreover, maintaining a healthy liver is vital for maximizing heart health. Nonalcoholic fatty liver disease (NAFLD), a growing epidemic, has been linked to increased heart disease risk. Popular fat-burning products injure the liver, which can be detrimental to cardiovascular health. Therefore, you are going to be introduced to resources that will enable you to identify products that can damage your liver and diminish your coronary health.

Additionally, key factors such as heart-healthy vitamins, the best food sources, superior vitamin formulations, and when to take supplements are discussed here. You will also discover corrections to common misconceptions. Additionally, daily supplementation schedules have been included for different age groups. Moreover, I go a step further by identifying several options to achieve the best quality for cost.

Please note that I have no financial interests in the products I recommend. My only interest is in sharing information to improve and extend your life.

References to "superfoods," magic diets, and mystical secrets from faraway lands are not contained in this book. However, you will discover a sustainable, common-sense approach to building and maintaining a strong and healthy heart. You will also be introduced to important terms that adults of all ages should know, such as *endothelial dysfunction* and *nocturnal blood pressure dipping*. As you read about these and other common yet rarely discussed conditions, you will begin to realize how easily you can lower your risk for heart disease, hypertension, stroke, obesity, and more.

When appropriately applied, vitamin therapy can transform your system into a full-time antagonist to common forms of heart disease, even while you sleep. Vitamin K2 is a prime example. Vitamin therapy also delivers an array of additional health benefits, including stronger bones, faster healing, greater endurance, and longevity. The more you read, the more you will appreciate the ease of control at your command over your personal health, fitness, and quality of life.

The information has not been cherry-picked to support foregone conclusions. Again, my goal is to show you a path of least resistance to superior heart function and overall health—a path you won't mind walking for the rest of your life.

YOUNG ADULTS

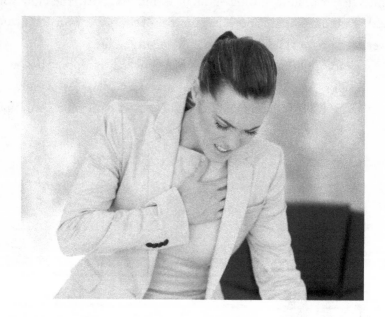

HEART HEALTH IS NOT A topic solely for individuals age forty and older; it is an important and exciting subject for us all.

Vitamin and mineral deficiencies rob your cardiovascular system of peak performance and can set the stage for hypertension, heart attack, or stroke. Additionally, a growing epidemic of obesity, sleep disorders, and nonalcoholic fatty liver disease (NAFLD) dramatically increases the risk of developing these and other life-threatening conditions.[1,2]

Now is the time to begin your journey toward maintaining a healthy liver, improved arteries, and a strong, vigorous heart.

HOW TO USE THIS BOOK

DUE TO THE COMPLEX NATURE of the cardiovascular system, *Heart Disease & Hypertension: Vitamin Therapy for a Healthy Heart* dives slightly deeper into medical terminology than my previous book. The more you understand the causes of heart disease, the more you will appreciate the power you have to prevent or reverse it.

It is essential to form a basic understanding of a few terms that you may be unfamiliar with, such as *endothelium, vascular smooth muscle,* and *vasodilation.* These and other critical components are part of your coronary arteries and their internal processes. Don't concern yourself with these "odd" sounding terms just yet, as they will be covered in greater detail within the following six chapters. As you begin to understand their roles, the solutions that follow will make sense.

Subsequent chapters will focus on the best nutrients and their sources to prevent or lessen common causes of heart disease. You will discover numerous peer-reviewed studies in which participants drastically reduced their risk for developing heart disease or reversed it to some extent. More importantly, they achieved these remarkable results by ingesting ordinary food, drinks, or supplements that are readily available at local grocery stores and vitamin retailers.

CHAPTER ONE

HEART DISEASE

HEART DISEASE—MORE ACCURATELY DEFINED AS *cardiovascular disease*—is a catch-all phrase encompassing a variety of heart-related conditions. One out of every four American deaths is caused by heart disease.[3] It is the number one killer of women and men in the USA and abroad. Well over half-a-million people die from heart disease each year in America alone. Although the subject can be quite complex, we will begin with a less complicated explanation.

Most of us are aware that blood flows through arteries and veins, otherwise known as blood vessels. The most common form of heart disease stems from partially obstructed coronary arteries, which overwork or starve the heart of oxygen and other vital substances. This condition is called *coronary artery disease (CAD).* As CAD progresses, heart muscle tissue can be permanently injured or even die. An obstruction develops when plaque builds up inside the arteries, narrowing the passageway, forcing the heart to work much harder. This additional force also increases blood pressure, causing hypertension.

To demonstrate this condition, place all four fingers on one hand together, side-by-side. Keep them together during this demonstration. Make a passageway (hole) by connecting the tip of your index finger with the end of your thumb. Press the side of your hand (thumb and index finger) around your lips and breathe through the passageway. You should now be breathing through your fingers and the palm of your hand. Do not perform the following step if it is not safe for you to do so.

Slowly make a fist, narrowing the passageway as you breathe. As the passageway narrows, notice the increase in pressure you must exert to push and pull the air through. Remove your hand. Decreasing the size of the hole simulates plaque building up inside of arteries. The heart must exert a similar level of additional pressure to push blood through constricted (narrowed) arteries each day without rest.

A full obstruction (embolism) completely blocks a specific area of an artery, like a clogged drain. A blockage occurs when a piece of plaque, blood clot, etc., breaks off and travels to a narrow passageway. Whatever section of the body that is normally fed by that obstructed vessel may quickly starve and die. The result is often a heart attack or stroke. Partially obstructed arteries increase the likelihood of a complete obstruction occurring because smaller objects can block these narrowed pathways.

As frightening as CAD may be, simple preventable measures will empower you to avoid and even reverse it, placing the odds of averting a heart attack heavily in your favor. For many, preventing heart disease and improving heart function is possible. Individuals who suffer from CAD can rebound from it and improve their quality of life.

Most people are aware that physical activity is important for building and maintaining a healthy heart. However, many individuals find it challenging to follow a rigid exercise regimen. Take comfort in knowing that a few dumbbells or resistance bands and a brisk, scenic walk are all the tools and activity you need. Dancing is also a great way to exercise.

Whether you exercise or not, nothing prevents you from enjoying a few heart-healthy substances. You are encouraged to think in terms of degrees. You do not have to choose between everything that may be good for your heart or nothing at all. Whatever you choose, do not succumb to the ideology of all or nothing. Anything you are willing to do to lower your risk is helpful. However, some choices have a greater impact than others.

CHAPTER TWO

YOUR MIRACULOUS HEART

INSIDE THE HUMAN BODY IS a vast network of flexible *pipes* called blood vessels. These vessels deliver life-giving blood to and from virtually every part of your body. Blood vessels, in conjunction with your heart, form the body's cardiovascular system. Your heart sets the pace to maintain the proper flow.

Blood carries oxygen, nutrients, protein, hormones, and disease-killing antibodies to various organs and tissues to keep you healthy, alert, and strong. Blood also carries waste products, including carbon dioxide, away from your body's cells for disposal. The heart is a specialized muscle that rapidly contracts and relaxes to provide tissue and cells the material and fuel they need to stay alive and to function properly.

BLOOD VESSELS

Blood vessels that make up the cardiovascular system come in three primary types—*arteries*, *veins*, and *capillaries*. Each type of vessel performs a different function.

- Arteries carry blood that is rich in oxygen away from the heart to body organs and tissues. The primary artery originating from the heart is known as the aorta. From here, arteries branch out into several smaller arteries as they carry nutrients and oxygen-rich blood to the rest of the body.
- Veins carry blood that is deficient in oxygen but high in waste products from the body to the heart. These waste products are designated to be excreted (removed) from the body. As veins approach the heart, they become larger in diameter.
- Capillaries are tiny vessels, much thinner than a human hair. They connect the veins to arteries.

Out of these blood vessels, *arteries* will be our primary focus for combatting heart disease. Individuals may not be aware that arteries are more than just hollow tubes. Amazingly, they are comprised of multiple layers, with each layer serving a specific purpose. Two layers of extreme interest are the *endothelium* and *vascular smooth muscle* (see Figure 1).

The endothelium is a thin, smooth, flexible layer of cells that make up the inner lining of your arteries. When healthy, endothelium protects the arteries from plaque buildup and stiffness and serves other vital functions.

Vascular smooth muscle surrounds the artery. This layer relaxes and contracts, adjusting the arteries' inner diameter to control blood flow, regulate temperature, and support other processes throughout the body.

Via key substances, individuals can help keep their arteries relaxed (dilated), smooth (nonstick), and flexible, resulting in lower blood pressure, improved circulation, preventing plaque buildup, and minimizing long-term heart strain.

Figure 1. Healthy Artery

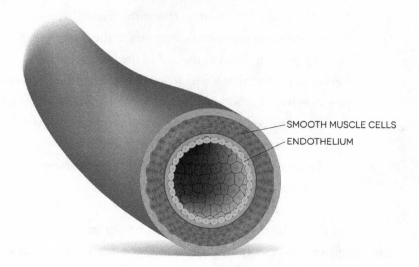

SMOOTH MUSCLE CELLS
ENDOTHELIUM

Cells that form the endothelium can become damaged, resulting in a harmful condition called endothelial dysfunction. Our strategy is to provide blood vessels the materials they need to maintain healthy endothelium and responsive, smooth vascular muscle. Doing so will drastically reduce your risk of developing heart disease and hypertension while improving your circulatory system's performance.

Endothelial dysfunction will be discussed in greater detail in subsequent chapters. Before doing so, it will be helpful to have a basic understanding of the heart. Pumping life-giving blood to sustain life is the heart's primary task. It accomplishes this momentous undertaking through three critical functions:

- Maintaining proper rhythm
- Maintaining healthy heart muscle
- Maintaining efficient blood flow

Your heart contains four chambers (sacks) that work collectively to refresh and circulate blood. The walls of your heart are made of specialized muscle tissue that contracts and relaxes to create the pumping effect. When the muscles relax, fresh oxygenated blood fills your heart. When these muscles contract, oxygen-rich blood is squeezed out of the heart through arteries to nourish and protect the body. Like all other muscle tissue, heart muscles need a constant supply of oxygen and nutrients. Therefore, the heart nourishes itself through the *coronary arteries*.[4]

Your heart maintains an efficient flow of blood through four specialized valves. Normal blood flow may be disrupted should any of these valves stop working correctly. Signs of heart valve issues include heart palpitations, chest pain or angina, and shortness of breath.

HEART ATTACK VS. CARDIAC ARREST

There is some confusion for many individuals over the difference between a *heart attack* and *cardiac arrest,* likely resulting from the terms often being used interchangeably. However, these are two different conditions with their own sets of implications. The former is associated with cutting off the blood supply to the heart. The latter is related to an interruption or change to the electrical signals controlling the heartbeat and its rhythm. The following chapters will provide a better understanding of the difference between these two occurrences.

CHAPTER THREE

HEART ATTACK

ACCORDING TO THE CDC, *735,000 Americans suffer a heart attack every year,* with nearly a third being people who have previously experienced one.[5]

A heart attack occurs when a blockage in the artery prevents the heart from receiving oxygen-rich blood. As discussed previously, such blockages typically occur when cholesterol-laden plaque in the lining of an artery ruptures, forming a clot. Therefore, a heart attack can be viewed as a plumbing problem, similar to a clogged pipe. Typically, when the blocked artery is not reopened quickly, the part of the heart that is usually nourished by the clogged artery starts to die. The sooner the blockage is removed and blood flow is restored, the less the damage caused.

Heart attack symptoms may include intense discomfort in the chest and other areas of the upper body, cold sweats, shortness of breath, and nausea or vomiting. These may be immediate or gradual, persisting for hours or days. Refer to The American Heart Association's website for more information.

The following image depicts stages of progression of coronary artery disease (CAD) from left (open passageway) to right (restricted passageway). The artery on the far left will provide higher blood flow volume with less pressure than the one on the far right. The artery on the right sets the stage for a complete blockage, resulting in a heart attack.

Figure 2. Coronary Artery Disease (CAD)

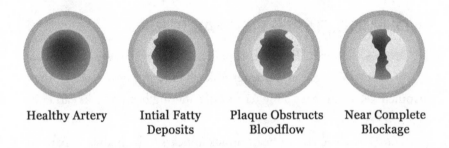

| Healthy Artery | Intial Fatty Deposits | Plaque Obstructs Bloodflow | Near Complete Blockage |

Figure 3. Heart Attack

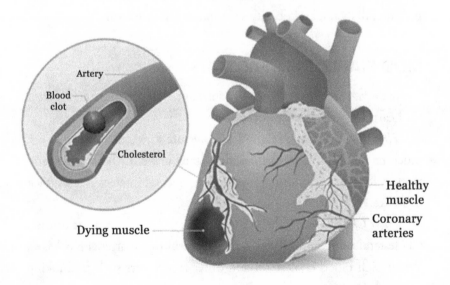

Fortunately, most people who suffer a heart attack survive. However, any form of heart attack, whether big or small, can permanently injure the heart or be fatal.

Thanks to extensive research, medical experts have identified several factors that increase a person's risk for heart attack. The more risk factors a person has, the greater the chances of suffering a heart attack. These risk factors can be broadly classified into three groups—non-modifiable, modifiable, and contributing risk factors.

NON-MODIFIABLE RISK FACTORS

Age: A majority of heart attack patients are above the age of sixty-five.

Gender: Men are at a greater risk of suffering heart attacks than women. Men also have a higher risk of suffering heart attacks earlier in life.

Ethnicity: The risk of heart attack appears to be higher in African Americans, Hispanics, and American Indians than Caucasians. According to a review published by *Harvard Health Publishing*, "these differences appear to stem from an increased prevalence of high blood pressure, diabetes, and obesity seen in some populations."[6]

MODIFIABLE RISK FACTORS

Smoking: Smoking tobacco is a substantial, independent risk factor for heart disease and heart attacks.

High Blood Pressure: High blood pressure forces the heart to work much harder. This continual workload may make the heart stiffer and thicker, leading to abnormal functioning and, ultimately, heart attack or stroke.

High Cholesterol: High cholesterol raises the risk of heart disease. Cholesterol waste tends to form plaque, resulting in arterial blockages. When high blood cholesterol and other risk factors such as smoking and high blood pressure exist in a person, heart attack risk increases dramatically.

Nonalcoholic Fatty Liver (NAFL): NAFL has been linked to an increased risk of cardiovascular disease.[7,8]

Obesity and Overweight: Excess body fat often results in high cholesterol and high blood pressure. These are major risk factors for heart disease, heart attack, and stroke.

Physical Inactivity: Lack of physical activity contributes to the formation of other risk factors such as high cholesterol, obesity, and diabetes.

Diabetes: Diabetes is yet another risk factor for heart attack. According to an article published by the American Heart Association, at least 68 percent of people with diabetes over sixty-five years of age die of some form of heart disease.[9]

CONTRIBUTING RISK FACTORS

Stress: Stress is a multifaceted and dynamic condition. There seems to be a relationship between heart attacks and the level of stress in a person's life. These are also unsurprisingly tied to unhealthy behaviors. For instance, stress may cause a person to fall into bad habits, such as smoking, not sleeping, and overeating, thus increasing heart disease risk.

Alcohol: Experts strongly advise against excessive drinking because it has been linked to cancer, stroke, and heart disease. The National Institute on Alcohol Abuse and Alcoholism suggests limiting drinking to no more than three fluid ounces per day.

Diet and Nutrition: A healthy diet rich in minerals, vitamins, fiber, and other micronutrients but lower in calories will help you control many of the risk factors for heart attacks, such as cholesterol, diabetes, weight, and blood pressure.

CHAPTER FOUR

CARDIAC ARREST

YOUR HEART HAS AN ELECTRICAL system that keeps it beating in a regular rhythm. Unlike a heart attack, cardiac arrest can occur suddenly as the heart unexpectedly stops beating. It is triggered by an electrical malfunction in the heart, which causes an irregular heartbeat (arrhythmia). A cardiac arrest is more of an electrical problem.

Electrical signals in your heart control the timing and organization of your heartbeats. When these electrical signals stop working properly, the heart's chambers beat in a chaotic and uncoordinated manner, or the heart may suddenly stop beating altogether. An electrical shock can cause cardiac arrest. More than *356,000 out-of-hospital cardiac arrests (OHCA) occur every year in the US alone. Of this number, 90 percent turn out to be fatal.*[10]

The standard treatment for cardiac arrest is to administer cardiopulmonary resuscitation (CPR) immediately. An electrical device called a defibrillator can be used to deliver a large electrical shock to jumpstart the heart's natural electrical signal.

CAUSES AND RISK FACTORS OF CARDIAC ARREST

Cardiac arrests are often common in people with underlying heart disease, prior heart attack, or some form of heart failure. There are several factors that can increase a person's risk of cardiac arrest. Two leading factors are:

- Previous heart attack
- Coronary artery disease (CAD)

At *least 75 percent of sudden cardiac arrest cases occurred in people who have previously suffered heart attacks.* There is a higher likelihood of suffering sudden cardiac arrest within the first six months after a heart attack.

Statistics have also shown that at least 80 percent of sudden cardiac arrest cases involved patients with CAD. This disease can be passed genetically or develop over time. Individuals who have suffered a prior episode of cardiac arrest are at greater risk of experiencing another event. Additional risk factors for cardiac arrest include having a family history containing one or more of the following conditions:

- Sudden cardiac arrest (SCD)
- Congenital heart defects
- Abnormal heart rhythms
- Parkinson-White syndrome
- Fainting without a known cause
- Obesity
- Diabetes

Steps that are taken to reduce the risk of having a heart attack will also reduce the risk of cardiac arrest due to the high correlation. These steps will also help prevent or reduce hypertension (high blood pressure).

CHAPTER FIVE

ENDOTHELIUM AND HEART HEALTH

AS PREVIOUSLY MENTIONED, *THE ENDOTHELIUM* is a collection of endothelial cells, forming a wall that lines the inside of your blood vessels (see Figure 1). One little-known fact is this exceedingly thin inner lining that most people have never heard of is a primary contributor to your heart health.[11]

The endothelium serves multiple roles and regulates many critical functions, such as inflammation and wound healing. Due to its extreme importance to heart health, endothelium health will be discussed periodically throughout this book. Maintaining healthy endothelial function is essential for protecting and strengthening the heart. Fortunately, maintaining and even healing this critical arterial lining is not difficult.

BLOOD PRESSURE CONTROL

The endothelium is only one cell thick. However, this ultra-thin lining causes arteries to contract and relax, allowing blood to flow at different pressures throughout the body. This fantastic ability impacts your blood pressure at rest and plays an active role during high-intensity activities, such as running, cycling, weight-lifting, dancing, and more. Moreover, increasing and restricting blood flow contributes significantly to regulating your body's temperature. A healthy endothelium is a major cornerstone for a healthy and active life.

PERMEABILITY FOR CELL TRANSPORTATION WHERE NEEDED

The endothelium also serves as a protective barrier, regulating the flow of elements into and out of the bloodstream. It can become permeable, allowing white blood cells to move into different parts of the body to protect the body from disease.

ENDOTHELIAL DYSFUNCTION

Regarding heart disease, the endothelium is extremely important to cardiovascular processes. When endothelial cells fail to function correctly, the condition is referred to as endothelial dysfunction. The dangers of endothelial dysfunction include:

- Hypertension (high blood pressure)
- Atherosclerosis (plaque buildup inside arteries)

If the endothelial walls constrict (narrow) too much, hypertension is a genuine concern. According to a 2014 article by the *Global Cardiology Science and Practice* journal, this condition significantly increases the risk of a heart attack.[12]

Many discussions regarding heart health revolve around cholesterol. However, endothelial dysfunction is a major contributor to the buildup of plaque inside arteries. Nitric oxide (NO) is essential for preventing molecules from sticking to the vessel walls, acting as an anti-inflammatory agent. Endothelial dysfunction manifests as endothelium cells failing to produce nitric oxide.[13] Diminished nitric oxide production allows molecules to *stick* to the walls and bind together to form plaque. Plaque narrows and stiffens arterial passageways, increasing the risk of cardiovascular events such as stroke or heart attack. This condition can be mitigated and reversed.

Figure 4. Endothelial Dysfunction Arterial Damage

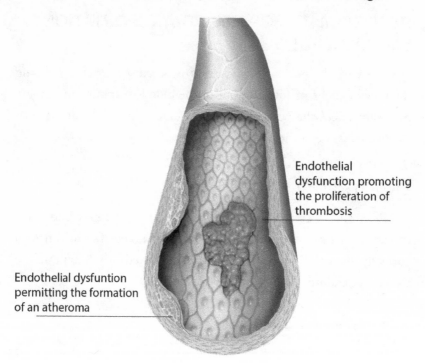

Endothelial dysfunction promoting the proliferation of thrombosis

Endothelial dysfuntion permitting the formation of an atheroma

Maintaining this vital inner lining's health and resiliency is often the missing link to heart disease prevention. Stopping and reversing endothelial dysfunction is synonymous with preventing and reversing common forms of cardiovascular disease—more awareness about the importance of this incredible inner lining is long overdue.

Nitric Oxide (NO) provides a broad range of health benefits for deterring heart disease, influencing healthy arterial processes, and maintaining proper endothelial function.[14,15] NO is a gas that is constantly produced within endothelial cells.

Diminished NO production is directly associated with several adverse conditions, such as diabetes, hypertension, and heart failure.[16,17] Therefore, supporting the natural production of NO within the endothelium is another integral component for preventing cardiovascular disease and improving circulation. Many of the vitamins, minerals, and plant-based substances discussed later can accomplish this for you.

Vasodilation is simply the internal widening of blood vessels. Blood vessels dilate (become more open) when smooth muscle surrounding them and the endothelium relax. As blood vessels widen, more blood flows with less force behind it, increasing circulation, lowering blood pressure, and reducing strain on the heart.

Vasodilation and vasoconstriction (narrowing of blood vessels) is a natural process regulated by the endothelium to control blood flow and body temperature. Endothelial dysfunction diminishes the ability to constrict and dilate blood vessels.

NO production, vasodilation, and vasoconstriction are critical functions regulated by the endothelium. For these and other reasons, such as preventing plaque buildup, maintaining a healthy endothelium is essential to maintaining a healthy heart.

Cholesterol is crucial for all animal life. Each of your cells produces cholesterol. Yet, most cholesterol is manufactured in your liver and intestines. Cholesterol comes in various degrees of density; two prominent forms are low-density lipoprotein (**LDL**), the bad stuff in excessive quantities, and high-density lipoprotein (**HDL**), the good stuff. High levels of LDL have been consistently linked to an increased risk of heart disease.

Healthy endothelium produces NO, which helps prevent LDL from sticking together to form clusters of plaque that can stiffen arteries and obstruct blood flow. LDL will be discussed in several of the following chapters.

It would be disingenuous of me to exclude a published review suggesting there is no correlation between high cholesterol levels and heart disease.[18] However, the consensus among many medical professionals concludes that there is indeed a definite correlation.

CHAPTER SIX

HYPERTENSION

WHEN YOUR HEART BEATS, IT contracts to pump blood through your vessels, then relaxes momentarily. Your arteries are under constant pressure in both states because they are filled with blood and other substances. When your heart contracts, arterial pressure spikes. When your heart relaxes, the pressure drops. This spike and drop are measured as *blood pressure*. The top number is **systolic blood pressure**, which is generated when your heart contracts. This is the high number. The bottom number is **diastolic blood pressure**, the pressure that remains when your heart is at rest. The following guidelines are current, but subject to change.

Normal (non-health-threatening) blood pressure is defined as measuring below 120/80, systolic over diastolic pressure. Although both numbers matter, systolic pressure (top number) is often the leading indicator regarding your arteries' health. The stiffer and narrower the arteries become, the higher the pressure.

Elevated blood pressure is defined as a consistent systolic reading of 120–129, while diastolic pressure remains normal, less than 80. If left unchecked, this condition may develop into *hypertension* (high blood pressure). It is common to have elevated blood pressure while engaged in high-intensity activity or under emotional duress. However, the pressure should eventually return to normal in healthy individuals.

Approximately *1.13 billion people throughout the world suffer from hypertension.*[19] More than 100 million men and women in the USA have hypertension or are taking medication to control it.[20] In 2018, hypertension was a primary cause or contributing factor in nearly half-a-million deaths in the United States alone.[21]

High blood pressure can have devastating effects on the body, such as heart attack, aneurysm, and heart failure. Hypertension is known as a silent killer. Many individuals aren't aware they have hypertension due to a lack of symptoms. The comparatively few people who do have symptoms may experience one or more of the following:

- Nosebleeds
- Severe headaches
- Fatigue or confusion
- Chest pain
- Difficulty breathing
- Irregular heartbeat

Hypertension Stage 1 occurs when systolic pressure reads 130–139, *or* when diastolic pressure reads 80–89, continually while an individual is at rest. At this point, your cardiovascular health is at risk because this rise in pressure is likely caused by restricted passageways (from plaque buildup) and hardened arteries. Your doctor will almost certainly prescribe dietary and lifestyle changes. Depending on your family and personal medical history, your doctor may also prescribe medications to lower the pressure.

Hypertension Stage 2 occurs when systolic pressure reads at or above 140, *and* when diastolic pressure reads at or above 90. The heart and arteries are not designed to function under these conditions continuously. Moreover, pressures this high are indicative of significant cardiovascular restriction and hardening. Your doctor will undoubtedly prescribe dietary and lifestyle changes, along with prescription medications.

Hypertensive Crisis occurs when systolic pressure reads at or above 180, *or* diastolic pressure reads at or above 120, *or* when both circumstances occur simultaneously. This condition requires immediate attention. Two categories of hypertensive crisis are *hypertensive urgency* and *hypertensive emergency*. Hypertensive urgency does not include symptoms, but hypertensive emergency does. Symptoms include chest pain, shortness of breath, altered vision, or difficulty speaking. Stroke, heart attack, or kidney damage can occur if the crisis is not addressed quickly.

Poor diet, unhealthy lifestyles, and excess weight put individuals at greater risk of developing hypertension. If left untreated, this condition can have detrimental consequences.

ATHEROSCLEROSIS

High blood pressure, over time, can damage the endothelium, resulting in endothelial dysfunction.[22,23] As discussed previously, this damaged area allows plaque to collect and build up in the arterial wall, restricting blood flow.[24]

ANEURYSM

Arteries that are constantly subjected to high blood pressure can weaken with time, resulting in a bulge (enlargement) in certain parts of the arterial wall. Such a bulge is called an aneurysm and more commonly occurs in the main artery, the aorta. An aneurysm can rupture, causing internal bleeding and death.[25]

LEFT VENTRICULAR HYPERTROPHY

The heart is a muscle. Like any muscular tissue constantly subjected to strong contraction and expansion motions, it thickens under high blood pressure. The left ventricle is the thickest chamber, and high blood pressure can cause further thickness—also known as *left ventricular hypertrophy*. This increases the risk of heart attack or heart failure.[26]

GOOD NEWS

These probable outcomes of hypertension are scary, as they should be. Fortunately, you will soon discover that high blood pressure can be prevented and even reversed, naturally. There are times when prescription drugs are the better option. However, far too often, they are viewed as the first and only option. Reversing deficiencies in readily available substances, such as magnesium and vitamin K2, can go a long way toward preventing and reversing hypertension.

At this writing, I am fifty-five years old with a family history of diabetes and hypertension. I have never followed a fad diet. I do not avoid gluten. Healthy carbohydrates are a regular part of my diet. I frequently consume grass-fed, organic (2 percent milk fat) cow's milk. I also do not chase after so-called *superfoods*. Over a period of three years, via vitamins, nutrition, and reducing stress in my life, I lowered my blood pressure from 120/77 to 113/73, on average. Consistency, reversing nutrient deficiencies, mitigating stress, and maintaining balance can lower blood pressure and do wonders for long-term health. Additionally, moderate exercise is an excellent habit to form for heart health.

Preventing or reversing hypertension walks together with preventing or reversing CAD, which drastically reduces your risk for heart attack, stroke, and sudden cardiac arrest. It also improves circulation, which delivers a host of added benefits.

CHAPTER SEVEN

MICRONUTRIENTS AND MISINFORMATION

VITAMIN AND MINERAL DEFICIENCIES ARE one of the greatest and most avoidable obstacles to maintaining heart health. Unfortunately, standard blood tests for certain nutrient levels are incredibly unreliable. Magnesium, which plays a significant role in endothelium and heart health, is one example.[27,28,29]

Nearly 50 percent of the magnesium in your body resides in your muscle and soft tissue. Just over 50 percent is stored inside of your bones. Less than 1 percent is contained in your blood. That minuscule amount often fluctuates due to everyday activities, such as a stressful day at work. Because of these and other reasons, blood tests conducted to determine magnesium levels are not reliable. The following table lists typical magnesium allocations in healthy individuals.[30]

Table 1. Measured Magnesium in Adults

Blood Serum + RBC	0.8 percent
Muscle + Soft Tissue	46.3 percent
Bone	52.9 percent

A magnesium deficiency will commonly manifest itself as muscle cramps, muscle twitches, fatigue, heart palpitations, and even cardiac arrhythmia.[31,32,33] In fact, these and other symptoms are common triggers for mineral blood tests. My blood tested negative for mineral deficiencies even after displaying severe muscle cramping and an unusual heartbeat.

When it comes to life-threatening conditions, you would be far better served by an early warning system. Several years ago, I found a doctor in the US who developed a more precise testing method according to the information provided.

The technical term for the procedure is *sublingual epithelial cell analysis*.[34,35] This testing method appears to be valid. The process used to collect cells for the test requires your doctor to take a mouth swab, similar to collecting a DNA sample. Your doctor sends the sample to a lab that uses analytical scanning electron microscopy and elemental X-ray analysis (EXA) to measure the mineral content inside your cells.

The results are reported as being so accurate that they are used to evaluate the ratio between mineral electrolytes within your cells. Test results include magnesium, calcium, potassium, phosphorus, sodium, and chloride concentrations. Knowing your doctor is involved in the process is reassuring. More details may be found at www.exatest.com.

Blood tests provide extremely useful information and are a powerful diagnostic tool. However, when it comes to the real danger of certain nutrient deficiencies impeding heart and artery function, the results can be very unreliable until you are acutely and chronically deficient.

VITAMIN THERAPY

Many dynamics influence your heart's health and strength, such as age, lifestyle, and genetics. One of the most manageable factors at your fingertips is vitamin therapy.

Numerous benefits can be gained from vitamin therapy. Vitamins and minerals that improve heart health also reduce the risk of developing a multitude of health problems. Wholesome food choices should be the first option for meeting nutritional needs. Vitamin and mineral supplementation should only be used to fill nutritional shortfalls.

Some supplement advocates recommend massive amounts of a single nutrient to achieve lofty outcomes. They discuss individual nutrients from a singular perspective versus as part of an overall system. My philosophy differs greatly from theirs.

Nutrients are synergetic. I liken them to a world-class symphony, in which every instrument and note must work in concert to deliver the best performance. Vitamins and minerals are more effective when they are in balance. Flooding your system with a single substance can cause more harm than good. More isn't better—*balance* is. I explain my views on this quite extensively throughout the book.

For instance, regular consumption of green tea can provide a variety of health benefits. However, supplemental forms of green tea extract, which are highly concentrated, have resulted in severe liver damage. Hence, an entire chapter is dedicated to supplement abuse and why you should avoid it.

GETTING STARTED

My first suggestion regarding supplements is to stop purchasing them from the grocery or drugstores with one or two exceptions. When considering your health and longevity, you are encouraged to invest in vitamin products seldom found in your local grocery store. Multivitamins are a prime example.

Instead, purchase products from an actual vitamin store or directly from the manufacturer's website. This is where you will find vitamins and minerals with a significantly higher level of quality. I have provided several manufacturers and product options for you to choose from throughout the book. However, you will find a complete list in Chapter 24 Daily Supplement Schedules.

My second suggestion is to be vigilant when purchasing vitamins through third-party internet retailers. One is especially known for offering free two-day shipping. The problem is not with the retailer. Instead, there are issues with some of the sellers who market to consumers through them. There have been instances of sellers shipping counterfeit or expired products. This does not happen often, but it does happen frequently enough to warrant concern.

If you choose to purchase online through third-party retailers, read the reviews for the seller. Examine the product upon arrival, and note the expiration date. Some sellers have even stooped to covering expiration dates with barcode labels. Do not become frightened or overly cautious, but do be careful.

Finally, formulations matter! For instance, supplemental magnesium oxide is barely absorbed into your system. In contrast, magnesium citrate and magnesium glycinate have far superior absorption rates, also referred to as a *high bioavailability rate.* The following chapters will clearly identify food sources and vitamin formulations with higher rates of bioavailability.

Now that we've discussed heart disease and the cardiovascular system, let's turn our attention toward the myriad of solutions and preventive measures. Regular consumption of this first natural substance increased the lifespan of various nonhuman test subjects by as much as 25 percent. Not only is it great for your heart, but it also appears to impede certain types of cancer. Moreover, it is readily available, and you might genuinely enjoy the taste.

CHAPTER EIGHT

POMEGRANATE

Impacts: blood pressure, heart health, digestion, diabetes, mental health, protein synthesis, sleep disorders, osteoarthritis

FOR CENTURIES, THE POMEGRANATE HAS been viewed as beneficial to general health. In recent decades, it has also been linked to better cardiovascular health. Today, we now have a much clearer picture of the pomegranate's heart health benefits. As you proceed, try not to get too hung up on some of the technical terms. It is the overall concept that matters.

LOWERS BLOOD PRESSURE

Some individuals may recognize the term *ACE inhibitors,* especially if they suffer from hypertension (high blood pressure). *Angiotensin-converting enzyme (ACE)* is a naturally occurring substance inside the body that influences blood pressure. Too much ACE causes blood vessels to constrict, which, in turn, increases blood pressure. ACE inhibitors are prescribed to counteract this effect. Remarkably, pomegranate juice has been demonstrated to impede the activity of serum ACE.[36] Researchers found that regular consumption of pomegranate juice reduces both systolic (top number) and diastolic (bottom number) blood pressures. They even recommended that the pomegranate be included in the established list of heart-healthy foods.[37]

IMPROVES ENDOTHELIAL FUNCTION

Pomegranate contains naturally occurring substances known as punicalagins. One of the striking characteristics they are known for is the stimulation of nitric oxide (NO) production. As previously discussed, NO acts as a vasodilator for blood vessels, hence improving circulation. It also helps prevent plaque from forming clusters and sticking to interior arterial walls.

According to the Catalan Institute of Cardiovascular Sciences, the metabolism of pomegranate leads to an extremely beneficial process called endothelial nitric oxide synthase, which relaxes blood vessels. It also promotes a significant reduction of inflammation markers along the blood vessels.[38]

LOWERS BLOOD CHOLESTEROL

Pomegranate has also shown promising results in lowering blood cholesterol, particularly in people with type II diabetes. During an eight-week period, diet assessments of individuals with type II diabetes were observed, and the participants' blood profiles were regularly evaluated. Concentrated pomegranate juice reduced LDL cholesterol.[39]

INHIBITS ATHEROMA

Pomegranate inhibits the clustering (sticking together) of LDL cholesterol, thereby preventing the development of atheromas in healthy individuals.[40] Atheroma are lesions of fatty nodules (see Figure 4) that collect on the arteries' inner lining. The nodules obstruct arteries, injure the impacted area, and stiffen the artery. Often, the first symptom is a heart attack.[41]

Rather than waiting for a heart attack to occur, regular consumption of a few ounces of pomegranate (fruit or juice) can pay far more dividends than a pound of *cure*. Given that it may lower blood pressure, it is wise to consult your doctor if you are taking any blood pressure medication.

SUPPORTS TESTOSTERONE

Pomegranate appears to increase testosterone levels and improves sperm quality. Over a period of two weeks, sixty male and female subjects ingested pure pomegranate juice while having their testosterone levels tested via saliva multiple times a day. On average, the men and women who participated in the study measured a 24 percent increase in testosterone.[42]

Moreover, the participants' systolic blood pressures decreased, on average, from nearly 123.7 to roughly 119.6, and diastolic blood pressures fell from approximately 74.9 to roughly 72.4. Similar research on albino rats indicated a noticeable improvement in sperm quality and density resulting from pomegranate juice consumption.[43,44]

There is some debate over potential side effects of testosterone replacement therapy, especially if not administered properly. However, naturally occurring, healthy testosterone levels support weight loss, muscle density, and lowers LDL cholesterol. All of which are good for the heart.[45,46]

The full extent of heart-health benefits of pomegranate juice is yet to be determined. However, there is compelling scientific evidence that shows it promotes cardiovascular health.

BRANDS TO CONSIDER

Natural, freshly pressed pomegranate juice is tart and somewhat sour. Two brands I often recommend are R.W. KNUDSEN, and LAKEWOOD. Neither brand is made from concentrate. I often find both brands in the organic section of various grocery stores. They are usually not refrigerated. If you examine a bottle closely, you may find a layer of sediment in the bottom of the glass, which is derived from the actual fruit.

Individuals who have never tasted freshly pressed, all-natural pomegranate juice should prepare to pucker up. The taste will be surprising as it isn't super-sweet, like the more familiar brand. One typically would not drink a full glass of all-natural pomegranate juice. Three to six ounces is more in line with a typical serving, which makes one bottle go a long way.

Consider drinking one small glass of pomegranate juice at least every other day, albeit every day may yield faster benefits. When combined with red grapes and green tea as part of a weekly regimen, missing several days should not be an issue.

CHAPTER NINE

GRAPES, WINE, AND RESVERATROL

Impacts: blood pressure, heart health, weight loss, anti-aging, mental health, cancer

AS WE EXPLORE MANY OF the essential micronutrients that can't be manufactured in the body, we must also delve into an incredible family of naturally occurring plant-based substances called polyphenols. Polyphenols come in various chemical formations that a growing body of evidence suggests provide a multitude of health benefits. More than 8,000 polyphenolic compounds have been discovered in a variety of plant species.[47] The one that we will focus our attention on is *resveratrol.*

Resveratrol, a powerful heart-healthy agent, is one of the primary reasons a glass of red wine is considered to be good for the heart. Resveratrol is a plant's chemical defense against predators and disease. It is created and secreted by plants as a natural response to harm, injury, or attack by external threats, such as bacteria, fungi, or pathogens. A leading source of this potent agent is the skin of red, purple, and black grapes.

In the human body, resveratrol is surprisingly beneficial. Research has shown this naturally occurring substance to accomplish amazing things, such as slowing cognitive decline and protecting the brain from damage. It also protects cartilage, preventing or relieving joint pain.[48] So what does a bit of resveratrol have in store for heart health?

ENDOTHELIAL SUPPORT

Previously discussed was the critical importance of maintaining a healthy endothelium to preserve cardiovascular health. As a reminder, the endothelium is the inner lining of your arteries and veins. Endothelial dysfunction is a condition in which the endothelium lining is not functioning properly, placing the individual at a much greater risk of hypertension and cardiovascular disease.

Although endothelial dysfunction is preventable and reversible in many cases, it is a leading cause of arterial wall stiffness and blockage impacting blood flow to the heart. A 2017 clinical study published in the *International Heart Journal* found resveratrol significantly reduced stiffness in the arteries, specifically the endothelial cells.[49] A 100-mg resveratrol tablet was administered to the participants each day for twelve weeks.

In a similar study, participants were given 100 mg of resveratrol daily for two weeks, followed by 300 mg daily for two weeks. Some participants received a placebo. Resveratrol increased activity that produces proteins to reverse arterial stiffness.[50]

BLOOD PRESSURE REGULATION

Besides reducing arterial wall stiffness, resveratrol also stimulates vasodilation. As discussed previously, vasodilation occurs when the smooth muscle surrounding the blood vessels relax, allowing the passageway to widen. Vasodilation results in increased blood flow, delivering more nutrients and oxygen, and reduced blood pressure, lowering the risk for heart attack and stroke. Resveratrol stimulates the increased production of nitric oxide (NO). NO promotes vasodilation, which, in turn, relaxes the blood vessels to reduce pressure and improve circulation.[51]

REDUCTION OF INFLAMMATION

Chronic inflammation is almost always associated with damaged blood vessels. The lengthy irritation may promote plaque growth, restricting blood flow to the heart, leading to possible heart failure. A 2012 article in *The American Journal of Cardiology* noted that resveratrol consumption significantly improves inflammation by decreasing plasma levels that would cause inflammation when spiked.[52]

CHOLESTEROL LEVEL CONTROL

The buildup of LDL cholesterol can cause the buildup of plaque, resulting in heart diseases like atherosclerosis. According to a 2012 research article published in the journal, *Molecular Nutrition & Food Research*, resveratrol consumption decreased LDL cholesterol in the bloodstream.[53]

Resveratrol should be an essential part of your investment in heart health. You can find it in grapes, berries, and, to some extent, nuts. As with all chemical substances, when it comes to dosing, despite internet blogger hype, more is not better. This is especially true when it comes to liver health. Although some individuals may realize short-term benefits from overdosing on nutrients, maintaining a healthy balance is the best approach.

POTENTIAL DANGERS IN HIGH DOSES

There is evidence of health benefits being obtained from high doses of resveratrol. However, several studies reveal high doses of this compound can be detrimental to one's health. In the 2010 study, "Dose-Dependency of Resveratrol in Providing Health Benefits," high doses of resveratrol:[54]

- depresses cardiac function
- inhibits the synthesis of RNA, DNA, and protein

- causes structural chromosome abnormalities
- blocks cell proliferation
- decreases wound healing
- impairs endothelial cell growth
- causes angiogenesis in healthy tissue leading to cell death

To their credit, another group published findings contradicting their earlier conclusion that resveratrol was safe at high doses. During this ninety-day trial, participants, sixty-five years of age and older, were administered 300 mg resveratrol, 1,000 mg resveratrol, and a placebo. Those who received 1000 mg showed a significant increase in the levels of coronary artery disease (CAD) risk biomarkers. No increase in CAD risk biomarkers was found in the participants who were administered 300 mg or given a placebo.[55]

Moreover, concerns have been raised on the potential impact of high doses on estrogen production. This is especially concerning for women who are at risk for various cancers.

Thousands of studies on this intriguing agent have been conducted. In one study, 10 mg of resveratrol was administered to individuals with coronary artery disease for three months, which resulted in improved heart function and endothelial function. It also reduced LDL cholesterol levels.[56]

NATURAL VERSUS SUPPLEMENTAL DOSE

To offer some perspective on naturally occurring levels versus the doses available in supplements, consider the following:

Naturally occurring doses of resveratrol from food and drink:

- Red wine (glass)—1 to 2 mg
- Red grapes (serving)—0.24 to 1.25 mg
- Red grape juice (glass)—0.17 to 1.30 mg
- Peanut butter—0.04 to 0.13 mg

Supplemental doses of resveratrol from various manufacturers:

- RESVERATROL-Maximum Strength Natural Formula 1,200 mg
- Trans-Resveratrol 1,000 mg
- Trans-Resveratrol 600 mg
- RESVERATROL 1,450 mg

HOW MUCH AND HOW OFTEN

Although mega-dosing on resveratrol may be enticing, my recommendation will always be consistency and balance versus overwhelming your system with any single nutrient.

Studies have seen great results with doses as low as 8 mg per day, with no apparent adverse effects up to 300 mg. Therefore, I do not recommend exceeding 300 mg per day for those who seek to supplement this agent. Numerous randomized studies measured significant benefits from low doses, with no adverse risks. In comparison, some high-dose trials have demonstrated similar benefits accompanied by considerable risk.

Consider the following age-related doses:

- Ages 20–34, 2 to 50 mg per day
- Ages 35–49, 2 to 100 mg per day
- Ages 50 and above, 2 to 200 mg per day

The ability to absorb nutrients diminishes with age. About 2 to 5 mg can be obtained by indulging in red grapes, real grape juice, or blueberries. Consider adding a mix of berries to a delicious, homemade smoothie. In doing so, not only will you obtain this powerful agent, but you will also receive much-needed fiber. If you are a red wine connoisseur, please drink in moderation.

Also, other substances offer similar benefits. Consequently, you can alternate your diet versus feeling 100 percent dependent on any single agent to achieve results. Missing a day or two should not be considered world-ending. Do not walk uphill through a hailstorm if you run out of grapes or supplements. A few days without should not be detrimental. If you feel the urge to supplement this compound, seek out the lower-concentrated doses. Also, consider taking it no more than four days per week, placing one or two days between doses. Mega-dosers, who claim to feel fine, may not have their liver or kidney enzymes tested regularly. By the time you *feel* liver damage, it's pretty extensive.

Consider eating red grapes or drinking real grape juice a few days per week. When combined with pomegranate and green tea as part of a weekly regimen, missing a week or two should not be an issue.

CHAPTER TEN

GREEN TEA CATECHINS

Impacts: blood pressure, heart health, bone health, weight loss, depression, diabetes, protein synthesis, nervous system, cancer

GREEN TEA IS CONSISTENTLY FEATURED in the list of the healthiest beverages in the world, and for good reason. It belongs to the Camellia family of plants and is loaded with antioxidants and flavonoids such as catechins. It has been hailed, for years, for its potential health benefits from fighting off infections to promoting general well-being. Recently, there has been an upsurge in experimental and clinical trials involving green tea—particularly catechins or epigallocatechin gallate (EGCG). EGCG is found in various plants, especially green tea. You will often see the terms *EGCG* and *catechin* used interchangeably.

Catechins are regarded as the most beneficial green tea components with antimicrobial, anti-inflammatory, and defensive properties against infections and adverse cardiovascular conditions.

ANTI-INFLAMMATORY PROPERTIES

Catechins can increase the production of specialized proteins that relieve inflammation.[57] Additionally, catechins' antioxidant properties may inhibit free radicals, reducing oxidative stress in your blood vessels.

Significant results via catechins include increased antioxidant enzyme activity and drastic improvements in cholesterol levels.[58] Additionally, a noticeable increase in the HDL (good cholesterol) to the LDL (bad cholesterol) ratio has been observed.[59] The anti-inflammatory and cholesterol impact of catechins substantially promotes a healthy functioning cardiovascular system.

CATECHINS PLAY A DEFENSIVE ROLE AGAINST CARDIOVASCULAR DISORDERS

Following their research, pharmacologists from the Rajendra Institute of Technology and Sciences stated catechins "have the ability to prevent atherosclerosis, hypertension, endothelial dysfunction, ischemic heart diseases, cardiomyopathy, cardiac hypertrophy and congestive heart failure." Catechins displayed the ability to decrease oxidative stress within cells and impede platelet clusters. Platelet clusters stick together and grow over time forming clots that can clog arteries. Preventing cluster formation has been proven to halt incidences of inflammation and blood clots within the cardiovascular system.[60,61]

POTENTIAL DANGERS

Unfortunately, advocates of mega-dosing have suggested that high doses of green tea extract are better for you than simply drinking green tea. They fail to realize that high doses of green tea extract resulted in moderate to severe liver damage in several individuals.[62] The associated term is *hepatotoxicity,* which stands for chemically induced liver damage.

Many popular fat-burning products utilize green tea extract as a primary agent. Studies have shown the detrimental effects of fat-burning products on the liver.[63] I strongly caution against ingesting high doses of green tea extract. Losing a few pounds on the front end is not worth damaging one of the most important organs in your body.

Conversely, the healthier your liver, the better your opportunity to lose weight and protect your heart. You will find more details on the importance of maintaining a healthy liver in Chapter 19 Liver Health.

To offer some perspective on naturally occurring levels versus supplemental doses, consider that many green tea extract products boast 1,000 mg of EGCG per dose. In contrast, an 8-ounce cup of green tea averages 30–100 mg of EGCG. Your liver is a critical gateway to general health. Protect it at all costs.

HEAVY METALS

Sadly, China, one of the largest tea-producing nations in the world, has the highest levels of lead in their tea. Additionally, popular low-cost brands in the USA have higher levels of lead and other metals stemming from tea imports.

Fortunately, most of the lead content is contained inside the leaves, and very little, if any, is released into the brewed fluid. *Do not chew, suck, or swallow the leaves.* Unfortunately, matcha tea requires drinking the ground leaves. If that tea is imported from China, consumers are ingesting lead and other harmful substances. The same is true of organic teas from that region.

Japanese tea has among the lowest lead content when compared to other tea exporters.

HOW MUCH AND HOW OFTEN

Although mega-dosing on EGCG may be enticing to some, two to four cups of green tea should work wonders for your heart and weight-loss goals. Loose leaf tea is often fresher than bagged tea and likely contains higher levels of healthy substances. Bagged tea is often more convenient.

I caution against supplementing green tea extracts containing more than 300 mg of EGCG per dose.[64] Fifty to 200 mg once or twice a day (several hours apart) may be safe for your liver. If you currently have a liver condition, consult with your doctor.

GREEN TEA TIPS

Green teas are often recommended to steep at 150–170°F for two to four minutes. Yet, some studies indicate temperatures near boiling release more catechins. Water boils at 212°F (100°C). One exhaustive study from 2019 resulted in peak catechin levels within green tea steeped at 203°F for ten minutes.[65] The difference was approximately 67 mg of catechins versus 58 mg in tea steeped at 140°F. Whichever temperature you choose, steeping five to ten minutes appears to release higher levels of catechins.

For optimum flavor, it has been suggested to add water before it comes to a full boil. I bring my water to a boil and allow it to cool for a minute or so. It has been suggested that drinking beverages at or above 149°F increases the risk of developing esophagus cancer.[66] The esophagus is a muscle-lined tube connecting your throat to your stomach. Allow tea to cool to a temperature that will not scald your throat or esophagus.

Regarding bagged tea, nothing prevents you from using more than one bag per cup. If you are an avid coffee drinker, you will likely lose two to five pounds just by switching to green or black tea. I lost four pounds in only two weeks after making the switch. Black teas are more oxidized than green tea, offering significantly lower levels of catechins. Habitual coffee drinkers may also consider substituting one or more cups of coffee per day with green tea.

CHAPTER ELEVEN

VITAMIN K2

Impacts: bone health, heart disease, arthritis, cancer, kidney stones, tooth decay

ALTHOUGH MORE TRIALS MAY BE needed, the preponderance of existing research strongly identifies vitamin K2 (a subcomponent of vitamin K) as a critical agent for maintaining a healthy heart.[67] Consuming just 100 mcg of this incredible nutrient per day can reduce the calcium in your arteries (where you don't want it) while infusing calcium into your bones and teeth (where you do want it). Simply put, K2 prevents both calcification (hardening) of the arteries and weakening of bones.

One of the most challenging aspects of taking this supplement is that, unlike zinc and magnesium, you will not feel rapid results. In time, you may wonder if taking K2 is a waste of effort and money. I assure you it is not. Have faith that taking vitamin K2 will yield extraordinary benefits and can extend your life. This fact is rooted in numerous studies conducted in several countries. Just because you don't feel a difference doesn't mean it is not working.

Vitamin K2 reduces a common form of heart disease by activating the matrix Gla protein (MGP).[68,69] This protein works by preventing calcium from building up inside the internal lining of your arteries. Therefore, the vessels in which blood flows to and from your heart will pass a higher volume of blood and be less susceptible to blockage. One study involving about 4,800 people found those who consumed higher amounts of vitamin K2 saw a 52 percent reduction in their risk of developing artery calcification. Moreover, they saw a 57 percent reduction in their risk of dying from heart disease! The study was conducted over a seven- to ten-year period. The daily intake for men and women was 30.8 mcg ± 18.0 and 27.0 mcg ± 15.1, respectively.[70] As demonstrated, massive doses were not required to realize measured results.

A three-year study published in 2015 concluded that prolonged use of MK-7, a naturally occurring form of vitamin K2, supplements reduces arterial stiffness in healthy postmenopausal women. Yet another study comprised of more than 16,000 women observed that participants with the highest intake of vitamin K2 had a much lower risk of heart disease. They also found heart disease risk decreased by 9 percent for every 10 mcg of K2 consumed per day. The daily intake of participants was only 29.1 mcg ± 12.8 mcg.[71]

Vitamin K2 also increases bone quality and density by activating a protein called **osteocalcin**. Osteocalcin is the *glue* that binds calcium and fresh material to your bone tissue.[72,73] Postmenopausal women were given vitamin K2 in its natural form of MK-7 over a three-year period. MK-7 reduced age-related decreases in bone mineral density (BMD).[74] In addition, MK-7 aided bone strength and significantly decreased the shrinkage in the participants' vertebrae.

VEGETARIANS

Vegans and vegetarians are at greater risk of developing a K2 deficiency. Fortunately, vitamin K2 is available as a supplement.

HOW MUCH AND HOW OFTEN

Two available supplemental forms—MK-4 and MK-7—perform the same function. However, MK-7 remains in your blood serum for up to three days. Mk-4 dissipates in less than a day. MK-4 requires higher doses to achieve similar results obtained through relatively low amounts of MK-7. For these reasons and more, I view MK-7 as the better option for supplementation.

The total daily adequate intake (AI) for naturally occurring K2 is 90 mcg (micrograms) for women and 120 mcg for men. Studies concluded that a higher intake of K2 resulted in lower mortality rates.[75] I do not endorse exceeding 250 mcg MK-7 or 5 mg of MK-4 in supplemental form per day unless directed to do so by a health-care professional. Moreover, it is perfectly fine to miss a day or two of MK-7 supplementation since a single dose remains active in your system for up to three days. You require very little vitamin K2 for optimal bone and cardiovascular health. Don't abuse it.

Here's a tip: It is difficult for individuals to determine the effectiveness of K2 supplementation. Rather than placing faith in one manufacturer, you might consider taking two different reputable brands. Either take them both daily or alternate between them every other day or week. If this is a bit confusing, stick with a single brand you trust. Just make sure it is a reputable one. Always remember that *popular* does not necessarily equate to *reputable*.

Table 2. Vitamin K2—Food

Food Type and Quantity	How Often
Natto (fermented soybeans) Head cheese Soft cheese Egg yolks Chicken breasts Chicken livers	One serving of any of these food items, once or twice per day, four to seven days per week Always consider calories and fat intake.

Table 3. Vitamin K2—Supplement

Suggested Supplement Options	How Much and How Often
Jarrow Formulas—MK-7 (90 mcg) Sports Research—MK-7 (100 mcg) Now Foods—MK-7 (100 mcg)	90–200 mcg (micrograms) four to six days per week. Or a combination of foods (listed above) and supplements.

ABSORPTION INHIBITORS

Broad-spectrum antibiotics and medications used to lower cholesterol interfere with vitamin K. Excess vitamin A also inhibits vitamin K absorption. K2 is a subcomponent of vitamin K.

ABSORPTION ENHANCERS

Vitamin K2 is a fat-soluble nutrient. Taking a K2 supplement with a fatty meal may improve its absorption. Foods with healthy fats, such as eggs (cage-free), flaxseed (oil or milled), avocados, olive oil, lake herring, lake trout, mackerel, wild salmon, sardines, and tuna, are a few options to consider.

BEST FORMULATION

- MK-7

LISTEN TO YOUR BODY

More research is needed to identify early symptoms of vitamin K2 deficiency and excess. Low bone density or teeth that are soft or easily fractured may indicate inadequate levels of K2. The challenge is that other nutrient shortfalls may also cause the same symptoms.

WARNING

If you take blood-thinning medications such as Warfarin, do not take vitamin K supplements without consulting with your physician. Taking vitamin D and calcium supplements without having adequate levels of K2 may increase your rate of arterial calcification. Balanced ratios are what your cells need to flourish.

TESTING

The importance of this nutrient recently entered the nutritional spotlight. Therefore, it may be some time before reliable, verifiable testing methods are developed to measure individuals' K2 levels.

It has been suggested that a vitamin K2 assay test may be worth considering. This test measures undercarboxylated osteocalcin as a functional marker of vitamin K2 levels. As discussed earlier, osteocalcin is the bone-binding protein activated by the presence of vitamin K2. Perform additional research and consult with your physician before subjecting yourself to this or any other tests. Several unreliable sources of information containing unproven scientific claims are hidden behind very impressive websites. Proceed with caution.

Due to K2's reported impact on arterial calcification, you may also consider a coronary calcium scan, which may provide some indication regarding the effectiveness of your chosen brand of K2 supplements.

According to the National Heart, Lung, and Blood Institute, the coronary calcium scan looks for specks of calcium in the walls of the coronary (heart) arteries. Calcifications in the coronary arteries are an early sign of coronary heart disease. As previously mentioned, K2 activates MGP (protein), which traps and removes calcium from your arteries. Therefore, a coronary calcium scan may provide some indication as to the effectiveness of the brand that is used or whether your diet alone is sufficient for your body's needs.

CHAPTER TWELVE

MAGNESIUM

Impacts: blood pressure, heart health, bone health, weight loss, depression, muscle cramps, menstrual cramps, diabetes, migraines, sleep disorders, fatigue, ADHD, kidney stones, nervous system, cancer

THE HEART IS ALMOST ENTIRELY composed of muscle. Muscle contractions and relaxations pump life-giving blood through a labyrinth of vessels within the body. Magnesium is one of your most powerful allies for sustaining and improving heart and blood vessel function. Unfortunately, magnesium deficiency is very common and has become a global phenomenon.

The *sodium-potassium pump* is an enzyme that generates electrical impulses to make your heartbeat. Magnesium is the primary component needed to regulate this process.[76]

Additionally, heartbeat contractions that create normal blood flow are generated through a symbiotic relationship between calcium and magnesium. When calcium enters the cells of the heart, its presence stimulates the muscles to contract. In contrast, the presence of magnesium stimulates the same muscle cells to relax.[77] Without the presence of magnesium, your muscle would not relax. Anyone who has suffered a severe muscle cramp has some idea of what this entails.

It is the competing relationship between these two minerals that results in a healthy heartbeat. As you may have already imagined, low magnesium levels can result in irregular or rapid heartbeats, which may be life threatening if left unchecked.

MAINTAINING NORMAL BLOOD PRESSURE

As mentioned, high blood pressure is a significant health concern affecting millions of people across the world. According to the Centers for Disease Control and Prevention, about 75 million adults have high blood pressure in America alone. In just 2014, high blood pressure was responsible for the death of more than 400,000 Americans through conditions like heart disease and stroke.

Magnesium has been found to be instrumental in reducing the risk of developing high blood pressure. Oral supplementation has proven invaluable to patients with hypertension, a condition where the blood is constantly at high pressure.[78] Several studies have found regularly taken doses of magnesium significantly reduces blood pressure, such as the one published in the *European Journal of Clinical Nutrition*.[79]

As discussed earlier, constriction of blood vessels contributes to increased blood pressure. Magnesium can help to relax blood vessels, allowing less-restrictive blood flow, and reducing stress on the heart.

PREVENTING ATHEROSCLEROSIS

Atherosclerosis, the condition in which the arteries' inner walls become clogged by the buildup of plaque, is extremely dangerous. In worse cases, the condition can even cause the rupturing of blood vessels when this clogging causes a blockage, and the building pressure tears a hole through the side of a vessel to escape.

Low magnesium levels have been linked to endothelial dysfunction.[80] Maintaining adequate levels of magnesium improves endothelial functions, inhibiting the development of plaque buildup inside arteries.

GENERAL HEALTH

As discussed in my previous book, *Osteoporosis & Osteopenia: Vitamin Therapy for Stronger Bones,* magnesium is the catalyst that enables you to effectively transform vitamin D3 from its dormant state into the active hormone. More than 300 processes that work to keep you alive and healthy require magnesium. Adequate (not excessive) magnesium intake is a common missing link to a properly functioning heart, optimum vitamin D levels, and overall better health.

Magnesium is necessary for many metabolic functions, including DNA synthesis, protein synthesis, and neurotransmission. Studies identify magnesium deficiency as a risk factor for various cancers, including breast cancer.[81,82] In addition, magnesium is beneficial for weight loss.[83]

Magnesium plays a significant role in heart health, having demonstrated positive effects on treating and preventing cardiovascular diseases.[84]

HOW MUCH AND HOW OFTEN

It is very challenging to obtain adequate amounts of magnesium through food and drink alone. Foods containing the highest concentrations, provide only about 20 percent of the recommended dietary allowance (RDA) per serving. Given the average American diet, many people may need to supplement at least 75 percent of their magnesium requirement to maintain adequate levels. The need for supplementation increases with high-intensity activities and age.

The RDA for magnesium is 310–320 mg (for women) and 400–420 mg (for men). Based on the tolerable upper intake level (UL), if you take 350 mg (or more) at one time, you may develop an upset stomach and diarrhea.

It is important to know the average person can only absorb up to 180 mg of magnesium per dose. To achieve good results, *do not take more than 200 mg at a time* because the rest will simply loosen your stool and pass through. One or two doses a day, with food, at 200 mg per dose, should meet the needs of most individuals. You can even break a 200 mg pill in half resulting in one 100 mg dose and a second dose at 200 mg, taken separately. For those who seek to perfect magnesium supplement absorption, some companies make 133 mg capsules. These can be taken two or three times a day, separately, for maximum absorption.

Table 4. Magnesium—Food

Food Type and Quantity	How Often
pumpkin seeds, 1 ounce almonds, dry roasted, 1 ounce spinach, boiled, ½ cup Swiss chard, 1 cup cashews, dry roasted, 1 ounce peanuts, oil roasted, ¼ cup black beans, cooked, ½ cup peanut butter, 2 tablespoons bread, whole wheat, 2 slices avocado, cubed, 1 cup	One serving of any of these food items, five to eight times a day, five to seven days per week. Always consider calories and fat intake.

Table 5. Magnesium—Supplement

Suggested Supplement Options	How Much and How Often
Swanson—Chelated Magnesium Bisglycinate (133 mg)	200–400 mg five to seven days per week. Or a combination of foods (listed above) and supplements.
Whole Foods 365—Magnesium Glycinate (~133 mg)	For maximum absorption, do not exceed 200 mg in a single dose. Do not take with calcium.
Now Foods—Magnesium Citrate (200 mg)	
Good State—Ionic (liquid) Magnesium (100 mg)	
Doctor's Best—Chelated Magnesium Glycinate (100 mg)	

ABSORPTION INHIBITORS

Calcium strongly inhibits the absorption of magnesium. Therefore, I do not recommend supplements that combine magnesium with calcium. Foods high in phytates or oxalates, such as grains, bran, unsprouted beans, soy, spinach, leafy greens, and nuts, inhibit magnesium absorption to some degree. Do not be overly concerned—you will still absorb some magnesium with these foods, just not the maximum amount. Alcoholic beverages, soda, stress, bleached sugar, intense workouts, and diabetes deplete the body's magnesium stores.

ABSORPTION ENHANCERS

Vitamin D enhances magnesium absorption. Complex carbohydrates, protein (other than soy), and medium-chain triglycerides (MCTs), such as coconut oil and palm oil, strengthen the intake of magnesium.

A quality formulation, such as magnesium glycinate, made by a reputable manufacturer, will absorb extremely well. Taking two or three doses—*at or less than 200 mg each*—will enable you to absorb much more magnesium than taking one large dose!

BEST FORMULATION

- Magnesium Glycinate (calming, relaxant effect that may aid sleep)
- Magnesium Citrate
- Magnesium Aspartate
- Magnesium Taurate
- Ionic (liquid) Magnesium

The formulations above are absorbed well. In contrast, the absorption rate of magnesium oxide is exceedingly low at approximately 4 percent. You will find that many popular multivitamin brands contain magnesium oxide; always check the nutrition label.

I commonly take Swanson Chelated Magnesium Bisglycinate (small capsules), KAL Magnesium Glycinate (The Vitamin Shoppe), and Whole Foods 365 Magnesium Glycinate (sold at convenient locations). Always read the nutrition label when purchasing supplements.

FORMULATIONS TO AVOID

The following formulations should be avoided. They are not harmful to you but offer diminished returns on your investment because they do not absorb well.

- **Magnesium oxide**—abysmal absorption rate. Very cheap to manufacture, which is why you will find it in several locations and formulations.

- **Magnesium complex**—here is where manufacturers often pull a fast one. Read the ingredients. *If magnesium oxide is one of the elements, do not purchase.* The label will often read "magnesium glycinate, magnesium aspartate, magnesium oxide." However, it usually does not stipulate the percentage of each type. Assume the majority of the product is comprised of magnesium oxide.

- **Calcium with magnesium**—Manufacturers may believe magnesium aids in the absorption of calcium inside your gut. Magnesium does, in fact, aid in the absorption of calcium. However, as discussed, this is achieved primarily by magnesium supporting the conversion process of vitamin D3 to the active hormone [1,25(OH)2 D] calcitriol. This conversion occurs inside your liver and kidneys, not inside of your gut. In fact, *calcium prevents magnesium absorption inside your gut* to a large extent. If your goal is to absorb magnesium, you *do not want to mix calcium with magnesium.* You will still absorb some, but not nearly as much as you would without including calcium. Protein may counter the effect of calcium's interference with magnesium absorption to some extent.

LISTEN TO YOUR BODY

Symptoms of magnesium deficiency include depression, anxiety, hypertension, muscle cramps, muscle knots, bone disorders, sensations of numbness or tingling, irregular heartbeat, loss of appetite, nausea, fatigue, sleep disorders, severe menstrual cramps, seizures, memory lapses, hallucinations, and disorientation.

You will probably not suffer all these things at once. However, if you suffer from any one or a combination of these symptoms, they may be caused or exacerbated by low magnesium. If you choose to supplement, do not go overboard.

If you are magnesium deficient, you should notice results within days, including but not limited to fewer muscle cramps, diminished menstrual cramps, and deeper sleep. Long-term effects often include improved heart function, improved blood pressure, better insulin regulation, stronger bones and teeth, and improved mineral utilization. Vitamin D levels and utilization should also improve.

You do not need excessive doses to achieve results. *Balance* is a primary factor for optimal mental and physical health.

WARNING

Typical effects of excessive magnesium intake include diarrhea and abdominal cramping.

TESTING

In many instances, blood tests can reveal a lot about your health. However, as discussed earlier, measuring blood serum magnesium levels is an unreliable method to identify a deficiency. The average person will likely display various symptoms resulting from long-term magnesium deficiency, such as frequent muscle spasms or even heart arrhythmia. Again, blood serum tests are typically used to verify a magnesium deficiency AFTER the onset of symptoms.

Soft tissue appears to be a better candidate for determining magnesium levels. Testing soft tissue is reportedly far more accurate for assessing mineral content. The previously discussed sublingual epithelial cell analysis (EXA test) can be initiated via www.exatest.com.

Methods for identifying a potential deficiency include:

- Recognizing symptoms (Listen to Your Body, above)
- Sublingual epithelial cell analysis (EXA test)

- Red blood cell magnesium test
- Diet assessment
- Urine excretion test
- Trial supplementation (Try 300–400 mg a day and note any changes. Best results occur by taking doses of 200 mg or less, two or three times per day, not to exceed 400 mg in a single day.)

You are encouraged to perform additional research and to consult with your physician before subjecting yourself to any procedure.

Find in-depth facts on myths and misinformation regarding vitamin D and the best method to remedy vitamin D deficiency in my book *Osteoporosis & Osteopenia: Vitamin Therapy for Stronger Bones.*

CHAPTER THIRTEEN

ZINC

Impacts: progesterone, bone health, thyroid function, weight loss, hair health, cholesterol, immune system, libido, depression, healing, seizures, asthma, ADHD, macular degeneration, acne

MANY INDIVIDUALS—ESPECIALLY THOSE OVER THE age of forty—are zinc deficient to some degree. Even a mild deficiency can significantly impact many aspects of your health, including heart health. The human body can't produce zinc on its own. For the body, zinc is essential for growth and development, tissue healing, immune system improvement, and so much more.[85] What does zinc do for the heart?

HEARTBEAT REGULATION

In the previous chapter, we explored how magnesium actively regulates the heartbeat via its unique relationship with calcium, which is essential to the entire process.

In 2015, researchers discovered that zinc also interacts with calcium in the heartbeat regulation process.[86] Before calcium can enter the heart cells, it must first be released through special *gates*, scientifically referred to as type-2 ryanodine receptors. The researchers found a direct interaction between zinc and the receptors, adjusting the calcium levels as calcium is released. Envision a faucet with you adjusting the volume of water flow. This is essential because it prevents the release of too much calcium into the heart cells, which could cause potentially fatal heartbeat rhythm and rate problems. Think of zinc as the heart's calcium receptors' security checkpoint, preventing calcium from overwhelming your heart.

Low levels of zinc are associated with high mortality rates in individuals who suffer from heart failure. Zinc is a critical component for energy transfer and proper heart function.[87,88]

LESSENING INFLAMMATION

Oxidative stress occurs when there are far too many free radicals present in the body for antioxidants produced by your cells to counter them. Free radicals are byproducts (or waste) generated by cells as they perform necessary functions. At high levels, free radicals can cause oxidative stress, which in turn results in chronic inflammation.

Temporary inflammation is actually beneficial because it serves a critical role in the immune response to injuries and infection. In contrast, chronic inflammation has been linked with several life-threatening conditions, including cardiovascular disease.[89] Zinc has impressive properties that have been found to effectively reduce oxidative stress.[90] As you may expect, fighting oxidative stress suppresses chronic inflammation, which supports keeping the heart safe from illness and complications. Other organs also benefit from this.

Individuals with cardiovascular complications such as cardiac ischemia, atherosclerosis, and even coronary heart disease presented low zinc levels in multiple studies.[91,92,93,94] Zinc proves to be an integral part of maintaining the cells of the heart and modulating blood flow functions that make it possible to maintain overall cardiovascular health.[95]

Studies have also found zinc supplementation prevented or impeded other conditions such as age-related macular degeneration

(AMD), incidences of infections, and more. Maintaining appropriate zinc levels has been shown to prevent bone loss and increase bone mass.[96] Zinc is also an important cofactor in vitamin D absorption.

Additionally, zinc deficiency lowers testosterone. Low testosterone levels have been linked to higher incidents of plaque in coronary arteries and increased risk of heart disease. Also, testosterone supports the production of nitric oxide and other components for endothelial health and repair.

An added benefit of resolving a zinc deficiency is the nearly instantaneous relief from some forms of erectile dysfunction. Just 10–15 mg of high-quality zinc taken with the last meal of the day will yield astonishing results for some individuals suffering from erectile dysfunction. Men in their forties and beyond will wake up like teenagers again, especially if a little boron (2–4 mg) is taken for seven consecutive days every other week. This will, of course, not work for everyone. To a lesser extent, women may also notice a heightened libido within a week or two of additional zinc intake.

Zinc plays a critical role in maintaining your immune system, along with your metabolism, thyroid health, mood, ability to heal, and more. Zinc levels decline as we age, compromising immune function.[97] Low zinc levels have also been linked to diabetes.[98] In turn, these functions directly affect your weight, blood pressure, energy, and sex drive. All of this plays a direct or indirect role in heart health.

Retinal zinc concentrations decline as we age, which may affect eye health. The human brain contains the highest amount of zinc. Low blood serum zinc levels have been detected in people suffering from depression.[99] In addition, the intensity of depression appears to correlate with the degree of zinc deficiency. Depression can have a secondary effect on heart health, stemming from a lack of motivation and energy.

Zinc imbalance can also result in heightened aggression or violence. Elevated levels of copper can result from a zinc deficiency, triggering neurological disorders. Also, a lack of zinc can contribute to neuronal injury or death.

Remarkably, a thirty-day supplementation of zinc gluconate resulted in a notable reduction in weight and BMI indices, according to a 2013 research article in the *Advanced Pharmaceutical Bulletin.*[100] Zinc is an incredible substance that goes far beyond impeding the common cold. Maintaining proper zinc levels is integral to heart health, lowers risk factors for additional health issues, and can improve the overall quality of one's life.

As we develop our understanding of how pomegranate, red grapes, green tea, zinc, K2, and magnesium support heart function and protect arteries from disease, we also begin to generate our road map to developing a healthier heart.

This simple approach is not rooted in speculation, superfoods, or wonder diets. Data has not been cherry-picked to support foregone conclusions. Information presented is rooted in an avalanche of peer-reviewed science, conducted in multiple studies around the world. More importantly, virtually anyone can follow these steps and achieve remarkable results for their heart. We have more ground to cover. However, it is helpful to construct a road map along the way.

VEGETARIANS

The bioavailability (rate of absorption) of zinc from vegetarian diets is lower than from nonvegetarian foods.[101] Zinc contained in meat absorbs exceptionally well. In addition, vegetarians eat larger portions of foods that contain phytate. Phytate binds minerals such as zinc and strongly inhibits absorption. Vegetarians may require up to 50 percent more zinc than nonvegetarians to maintain adequate levels.

HOW MUCH AND HOW OFTEN

Zinc is an essential trace element. Our bodies do not store zinc for long, which is why you need a fresh supply fairly often. Fortunately, you only need a little to achieve optimal cellular performance. The

Recommended Dietary Allowance (RDA) for zinc is 11 mg for men and 8 mg for women. The daily tolerable upper intake level (UL) is 40 mg for men and women. I alternate between 11 mg and 15 mg four days per week. The 15 mg capsule also contains 1 mg of copper. I break a 22 mg tablet in half for an approximate 11 mg dose.

If you are mildly to moderately zinc deficient and increase your daily intake, you may begin to notice results in just a few days. Results may include a stronger libido, leaner muscle tone, and better performance at the gym. Long-term results will include enhanced vitamin D utilization, faster healing of injuries, fewer illnesses, and healthier skin. Due to zinc's short shelf life within our system, consider eating zinc-rich foods or taking low-dose supplements three to five days per week.

Do not mega-dose on zinc. Studies have shown that excessive zinc intake can cause a variety of neurological and physiological problems, including high blood pressure. Daily zinc intake of 40 mg or more can result in copper deficiency. Lower doses of zinc do not appear to diminish copper absorption. If you do not tolerate zinc well on an empty stomach, take it with a meal or try a different type.

High levels of zinc can also result in hair loss. Several zinc supplements are sold in 30 mg doses, which is a bit high if taken daily. If you purchase 30 mg tablets, consider taking the full dose only two or three days per week (Monday, Wednesday, Friday), or breaking the tablet in half to take three to five days per week. The goal is to attain mineral balance.

Table 6. Zinc—Food

Food Type and Quantity	How Often
oysters, cooked (3 ounces)	Twice per week.
beef chuck roast, braised (3 ounces) crab, Alaska king, cooked (3 ounces) beef patty, broiled (3 ounces) breakfast cereal, fortified with 25 percent of the DV for zinc (¾ cup serving)	One serving of any of these food items, once or twice per day, four to seven days per week. Always consider calories and fat intake.

Table 7. Zinc—Supplement

Suggested Supplement Options	How Much and How Often
Jarrow Formulas—Zinc Balance: Zinc (15 mg) Copper (1 mg) Swanson—Zinc orotate (10 mg) Liquid Ionic Zinc (various vendors)—(10 drops = 15 mg) Whole Foods 365—Zinc (15 mg) copper (1 mg) Solgar—Zinc picolinate (22 mg)	Four to six days per week. Or a combination of foods (listed above) and supplements. Five drops of ionic zinc three to five days per week can be considered for children.
Pure Encapsulations—Zinc 30: Zinc picolinate (30 mg) Kal—Zinc orotate (30 mg)	Three to five days per week. Excessive zinc depletes other minerals and may cause psychological problems.

ABSORPTION INHIBITORS

Phytate—present in foods such as cereals, corn, and rice—inhibits zinc absorption to some degree. If taken together with zinc, iron or calcium supplements can have an adverse effect on zinc absorption. No impact on zinc bioavailability appears to occur from naturally occurring iron, such as found within red meat. Some medications, such as antibiotics and diuretics, can also inhibit zinc absorption.

ABSORPTION ENHANCERS

Meat-based protein such as beef, turkey, chicken, eggs, and seafood enhance zinc absorption. These foods also help to counteract absorption inhibitors.

BEST FORMULATION

- Zinc orotate (absorbs exceptionally well; not easily impaired by phytate)
- Zinc monomethionine (absorbs extremely well; not easily impaired by phytate)
- Zinc picolinate (absorbs extremely well; may irritate an empty stomach)
- Zinc citrate (absorbs well; may irritate an empty stomach)
- Zinc gluconate (absorbs well; may irritate an empty stomach)
- Zinc Balance consists of 15 mg of chelated zinc monomethionine and 1 mg of copper in a popular formulation called Opti-Zinc
- Ionic (liquid) zinc

LISTEN TO YOUR BODY

Symptoms of zinc deficiency can be easily misinterpreted or misdiagnosed. A compromised immune system resulting in frequent coughs or colds, sinus or respiratory infections, slow healing, or fatigue may be due to zinc deficiency. Mood swings, depression, ADHD, and difficulties with learning may also be symptoms of zinc deficiency. Zinc deficiency can also result in low testosterone or diminished thyroid function, which, in turn, can cause associated issues.

Very high levels of zinc can result in hair loss, nausea, vomiting, loss of appetite, diarrhea, abdominal cramps, and headaches. Mega-dosing on zinc will cause mineral imbalances, triggering mental and physical health problems. Additionally, excessive zinc can cause hypertension (high blood pressure).

Again, zinc supplementation taken with an evening meal or snack will enhance libido within an hour for the remainder of the night. This applies to men and women. However, as tempting as it may become, do not take excessive amounts of zinc.

WARNING

High-dose zinc intake significantly inhibits copper absorption and mildly inhibits iron absorption. You may also wish to consider slightly increasing iron intake via food or periodic supplementation when increasing zinc intake. Iron supplementation can be extremely hazardous and should not be taken lightly. Consult with your physician.

TESTING

- A zinc taste test may be an indicator of chronic zinc deficiency. Zinc sulfate is tasted, and your doctor will consider your response. It is convenient yet very subjective.
- A zinc serum test is more conventional. Unfortunately, several factors can cause inaccurate results.
- Blood plasma can offer an estimate of zinc levels in tissue. Cell levels are more useful as a measure of zinc nutritional status.
- Trial zinc supplementation at doses of 12–25 mg, four to five days per week, for a period of four to six weeks may reveal an existing zinc deficiency.

CHAPTER FOURTEEN

OMEGA-3 FATTY ACID

Impacts: heart disease, bone disease, arthritis, cancer, kidney stones, tooth decay

WHEN IT COMES TO MAINTAINING or improving heart health, omega-3 fatty acids should be at the top of your list.

Some consumers underestimate the unquestionable health benefits of omega-3 fatty acids. Individuals may never know the full extent to which omega-3 prevented them from having a heart attack and extending their lives (unless one could go into a parallel universe and see what their life would have been like without omega-3 in their diet). Thousands of studies have demonstrated the litany of health benefits garnered from omega-3 fatty acids.

Omega-3 fatty acids come in various dietary forms: docosahexaenoic acid (DHA), docosapentaenoic acid (DPA), eicosapentaenoic acid (EPA), and alpha-linolenic acid (ALA). Of the four, the human body utilizes DHA, DPA, and EPA. However, ALA, a plant-based omega 3, cannot be utilized until your body converts it to EPA, which has been shown to be extremely inefficient.

ALA can be converted into EPA and then to DHA. However, the conversion (which occurs primarily in the liver) is very limited, with reported rates of **less than 15 percent**. Therefore, obtaining EPA and DHA directly from foods and dietary supplements is the more practical way to increase levels of these fatty acids in the body.[102]

—National Institutes of Health

Omega-3 fatty acids are essential polyunsaturated fatty acids that are very useful in many body functions, including heart health, brain function, and regulating inflammation.[103] *Essential* nutrients, in this case, means the body requires them to function, but it is not able to make these nutrients on its own, thereby relying on dietary intake. *Nonessential* vitamins can be made internally via chemical processes.

Researchers around the world conclude that consumption of fish oil, which mostly contains omega-3 fatty acids, is associated with a significant reduction in heart disease. Moreover, a concentration-risk relationship has been identified. People who have up to 6.5 percent concentration of omega-3 fatty acids in the membranes of their red blood cells displayed a whopping 90 percent reduced risk of heart disease than individuals who have only 3.3 percent in theirs.[104] Similar results also demonstrate the cardio-protective effects of omega-3 fatty acids.[105,106]

TRIGLYCERIDES, LDL, AND HDL BENEFITS

Triglycerides are the most abundant form of fat in the human body. Major organs, such as your brain, heart, and others, use ketones for energy. Ketones are derived from triglycerides. However, in high quantities, triglycerides become detrimental to health and a risk factor for heart disease, stroke, and obesity, among others.[107]

Cholesterol, also a normal constituent of all body cells, including red blood cells, is a waxy fat-like substance that is involved in several biological processes. However, as discussed in previous chapters, excessive amounts can lead to the buildup of **atherosclerotic plaques** that stick to the artery walls causing coronary artery disease.[108]

Diets high in saturated fats and trans fats increase harmful cholesterol and triglyceride levels. In contrast, consuming foods rich in **polyunsaturated** and **monounsaturated** fats reduces heart disease risk and improves heart health.

Omega-3 (polyunsaturated) fatty acids benefit the heart by reducing triglyceride and LDL (bad cholesterol) levels while increasing that of HDL (good cholesterol).[109] Consumption of EPA and DHA in small doses (<1 g/day) has been shown to decrease the risk of death from coronary heart disease by keeping the heart muscle stable, reducing heart rate, and decreasing the risk of having abnormal heart rhythms (arrhythmias) such as atrial fibrillation. Cardiac societies recommend the use of EPA and DHA in reducing triglyceride levels.[110]

REDUCED ATHEROSCLEROSIS

Atherosclerotic plaques narrow and stiffen blood vessel passageways, thereby predisposing the individual to have ischemic (reduced oxygen) heart disease.

Intake of EPA and DHA enhances blood circulation and impedes vascular stiffness by reducing the ability to form plaques in the first place. These compounds also reduce the tendency of plaques to rupture. Embolic heart events have occurred when ruptured plaques are dislodged into the bloodstream and reach smaller blood vessels, which they occlude (clog), causing a heart attack.[111]

In a randomized control study carried out on patients about to undergo heart surgery, prior treatment with EPA and DHA led to changes in plaque structure, with stabilization of the plaques and no features of inflammation observed.[112] A stable plaque cluster is less likely to break off into the bloodstream and obstruct a blood vessel.

REDUCING BLOOD PRESSURE

High blood pressure is a major risk factor for heart disease. Chronic high blood pressure is associated with changes in the heart muscle's morphology and blood vessels. These changes predispose the individual to heart failure due to the excessive workload on the heart having to pump blood forcibly enough to overcome the high pressure in the systemic arteries.

Additionally, there is the associated endothelial (inner vessel lining) disruption that also predisposes individuals to atherosclerotic and coronary artery disease.[113] Ingestion of omega-3 fatty acids (especially EPA and DHA) effectively lowers resting blood pressure and enhances endothelial function.

Some other benefits of omega-3 fatty acids include reducing platelet aggregation and clotting tendencies, which are involved in ischemic heart disease (especially DHA), and a reduction of inflammatory markers that are implicated in the development of several chronic diseases (especially EPA).[114,115]

In addition to the heart benefits, research suggests omega-3 fatty acids help reduce symptoms of depression (both EPA and DHA, but especially the former), postmenopausal symptoms (EPA), and in vision and brain function. However, more findings are needed.

The role of omega-3 fatty acids in boosting heart health and preventing heart disease is uncontested. Most of the benefits ascribed to them come from the consumption of fatty fish and other seafood like salmon, sardine, tuna, mackerel, trout, shrimp, eel, sturgeon, etc., (EPA and DHA sources), and, to a lesser extent, plant foods like walnuts, flaxseed, soybeans, tofu, and some oils (ALA sources). Cardiac societies recommend a diet rich in omega-3 fatty acids (up to 1 g/day) for optimum cardiac health and function.

Your body can down-convert DHA to EPA, and up-convert EPA to DHA as needed. Baby formula manufacturers have been adding DHA to their products for nearly twenty years.

VEGETARIANS

Plant-based omega-3 occurs as ALA, which must be converted internally to EPA and then to DHA for use. Again, less than 15 percent of ALA consumed is converted within healthy individuals.

HOW MUCH AND HOW OFTEN

The total daily adequate intake (AI) for omega 3 is 1.1 grams (1,100 mg) for women and 1.6 grams (1,600 mg) for men. Although numerous omega-3 supplement options are available, seafood consumption is by far the best source.

It is worth noting that studies have raised safety concerns regarding fish consumption, such as farm-raised salmon containing low levels of mercury. Wild-caught salmon appears to be safer. Moreover, some data suggest diminished benefits of omega-3 supplements versus consuming seafood. Additionally, fish-oil supplements should meet third-party safety criteria, such as **International Fish Oil Standards (IFOS)** or **National Sanitary Foundation (NSF) Certified** for safety. Krill oil supplements may be more beneficial than fish oil but very cost-prohibitive for a similar dosage.

Table 8. Omega-3—Food

Food Type and Quantity	How Often
Salmon (4,100 mg) Mackerel (4,100 mg) *Cod liver oil (2,682 mg) Sardines (2,200 mg) Chia seeds (5,000 mg ALA) Walnuts (2,600 mg ALA) Soybeans (1,200 mg ALA)	One serving of any of these food items, two or three times per week. Always consider calories and fat intake. *NOTE: Cod liver oil also contains vitamins D and A. More than one tablespoon can raise vitamin A to levels that are detrimental to your health.

Table 9. Omega-3—Supplement

Suggested Supplement Options	How Much and How Often
Barlean's—Emulsified Fish Oil (1,500 mg) Transparent Labs—Krill Oil (500 mg) Sports Research—Fish Oil (1,250 mg) Dr. Tobias—Fish Oil (1,000 mg)	500–2,000 mg (micrograms) three to six days per week. Or a combination of foods (listed above) and supplements. NOTE: Dosage is listed per pill or tablespoon.

ABSORPTION INHIBITORS

Many fish oil supplements are in the synthetic form of ethyl-ester, which is reported far less absorbable than natural triglyceride formulations found in wild fish. Additionally, omega-3 fatty acids are readily destroyed by stomach acid.

ABSORPTION ENHANCERS

According to studies, emulsified fish oil absorbs better than encapsulated fish oil.[116,117] Additionally, enteric-coated capsules reportedly protect the contents from stomach acid and deliver it to the intestinal tract for absorption.

Taking an omega-3 supplement with a fatty meal may improve its absorption. Foods with healthy fats such as eggs (cage-free), flaxseed (oil or milled), avocados, and olive oil are a few options to consider.

However, the best source will be obtained via omega-3-rich protein, such as salmon and tuna.

CHAPTER FIFTEEN

IODINE

Impacts: metabolism, fatigue, depression, immune system, cancer, bone health, fibrosis, testosterone, cholesterol, coronary artery disease, autoimmune diseases, hair loss

IODINE IS ESSENTIAL FOR PROPER thyroid function. Maintaining optimum thyroid function is critical to many aspects of your physical and mental well-being, including heart health. This ripple effect is how we come to appreciate iodine's role in combating heart disease and other ailments.

The two overarching forms of improper thyroid function are **hypothyroidism** (a thyroid that does not produce enough thyroid hormone) and **hyperthyroidism** (a thyroid that produces excessive thyroid hormone). Hypothyroidism weakens the heart muscle and causes it to pump less forcefully. Consequently, people with iodine deficiencies are often found to have slow heart rates. Moreover, excessive iodine intake has been directly linked to hyperthyroidism, which makes the heart work harder. If left untreated, this can result in heart failure.

Iodine is a natural mineral that the body does not produce. However, it is essential to the normal body functions such as the production of thyroid hormones and the growth and development of the brain. Iodine is also used in medicine to treat certain kinds of infections.[118] Since the body cannot manufacture iodine, it is an absolute requirement in the diet. Some common foods that contain iodine include fish, dairy, vegetables, fruits, and iodized salt. What can iodine do for your heart?

BLOOD VESSEL DILATION

Thyroid hormones are also responsible for the dilation of numerous blood vessels throughout the body. Researchers at the Karolinska Institute in Sweden noted changes in body temperature sensitivities in the presence of excess and limited amounts of thyroid hormones.[119] Low levels of thyroid hormones had subjects feeling cold, while high levels resulted in them feeling warm. Coldness is due to the dilation of blood vessels, which lowers the body temperature, while the opposite remains true. Maintaining normal dilation capabilities in the blood vessels helps to regulate body temperature. Normal dilation also prevents blood-pressure-related heart complications.

The primary way in which iodine affects the heart itself and its subsidiary functions is through the influence asserted by the production of thyroid hormones. Having a diet that contains an adequate level of iodine is essential to normal heart function. Additionally, iodine is a natural cancer-fighting agent. Not only does it shrink cancer cells, it also causes **apoptosis** (automatic cell death) of some forms of cancer cells.

MYTHS AND MISINFORMATION

Even though the Recommended Dietary Allowance (RDA) for iodine is only 150 mcg (micrograms), some individuals ignited an iodine mega-dosing frenzy, suggesting supplementation of up to 12.5 mg (milligrams) per day. They suggest slowly increasing the dose to build a tolerance to their massive recommended amounts. The frenzy may be tied to a miscalculation within a 1967 research paper that focused on iodine consumption in Japan.

TRUTH AND REALITY

Virtually all credible data strongly cautions against consuming large amounts of iodine. The potential for exposure to a radiological hazard, such as the aftermath of a nuclear explosion, is the exception. Excessive iodine intake will cause your thyroid to decrease its iodine absorption and your kidneys to excrete more via urine. However, there are limits to how much excess iodine this self-protection mechanism can offset.

VEGETARIANS

Vegetarians and vegans are at greater risk of developing iodine deficiency. Soy and cruciferous vegetables such as broccoli and cauliflower interfere with the utilization of iodine.[120]

HOW MUCH AND HOW OFTEN

The RDA for iodine in adults is 150 mcg. The upper limit is approximately 1 mg (1,000 mcg). In the rare event of a radiological incident (such as a nuclear explosion), the CDC recommends a single dose of 130 mg of potassium iodide for adults under age forty.

Attaining proper iodine levels can yield both short- and long-term benefits. People who are moderately deficient may see results within a few weeks, including increased energy and weight loss. If you are not deficient, you may not feel any effects. Positive results may occur very gradually over several months for mild iodine deficiencies. Skipping a day or more of supplementation enhances the absorption rate. It sounds odd, but it's true.

China's National Iodine Deficiency Disorders Elimination Program decreased goiter rates among children from 20.4 percent to 8.8 percent in four years via iodized salt.[121] The International Council for the Control of Iodine Deficiency Disorders Global Network and the American Thyroid Association confirm that 150 mcg of iodine per day is adequate for most adults (except during pregnancy). [122,123]

Table 10. Iodine—Supplement

Food Type and Quantity	How Often
Sea vegetables Cod Turkey breast Eggs Milk Yogurt Cranberries Navy beans Potatoes (baked)	One serving of any of these items two or three times a day. Always consider calories and fat intake.

Table 11. Iodine—Supplement

Suggested Supplement Options	How Much and How Often
LL—Magnetic Clay Nascent Iodine - 1 oz. (400 mcg per drop)	One drop, one to two days per week
Go Nutrients—Iodine Edge Nascent Iodine (~300 mcg per drop)	One pill, three to four days per week
NOW—Kelp Caps (150 mcg)	(Or a combination of foods and supplements)

ABSORPTION INHIBITORS

Fluoride, chlorine, bromide (bromine, bromate), all of which are found in white flour, bread, rolls, soda, tap water, and most toothpaste products, inhibit the thyroid's ability to absorb iodine. Soy and cruciferous vegetables such as cabbage, broccoli, cauliflower, and brussels sprouts also interfere with iodine absorption as do caffeine products.

ABSORPTION ENHANCERS

Nascent (atomic) iodine absorbs exceptionally well on an empty stomach. Typically, the consumer must add a drop of liquid iodine to a glass of water and swallow. Nascent iodine can also be absorbed sublingually. It has been reported to be less toxic and better tolerated than other forms. There is no risk of heavy metals.

Molecular iodine supplements have grown popular and appear to absorb well on an empty stomach, and moderately well with food. Be advised that some forms of molecular iodine are sold in extremely high doses.

Potassium iodide is primarily absorbed within the gastrointestinal tract and is considered less effective than nascent iodine. Unless you have a properly diagnosed medical condition, a regimen of 150 to 250 mcg taken a few days per week should serve to maintain your thyroid health. Remember, you are also obtaining iodine from other sources. This is a supplement, not a replacement.

BEST FORMULATION

- Nascent (atomic) iodine (absorbs exceptionally well; superior form of iodine).
- Molecular iodine (absorbs well on an empty stomach).
- Potassium iodide (absorbs moderately well).
- Iodized salt is beneficial for maintaining proper iodine levels.

Unfortunately, too much salt may lead to other health issues, such as hypertension.

- LL's Magnetic Clay Nascent Iodine (atomic iodine) is highly effective.

LISTEN TO YOUR BODY

Iodine deficiency can cause impaired mental function, fatigue, goiter, or hypothyroidism (underactive thyroid). With hypothyroidism, you may feel colder and suffer memory lapses or even depression. Detailed symptoms are listed under Hashimoto's Disease on the following page.

Severe iodine deficiency during pregnancy can result in children with mental and growth disorders. Excessive iodine can cause hypothyroidism or hyperthyroidism (overactive thyroid), resulting in nervousness, irritability, anxiety, difficulty sleeping, perspiration, rapid heartbeat, hand tremors, brittle hair, and muscle fatigue.

WARNING

On June 5, 2013, the American Thyroid Association released a statement advising against the daily ingestion of iodine supplements in excess of 500 mcg.[124] They further stated that consuming more than 1,100 mcg of iodine per day may cause thyroid dysfunction.

Long-term exposure to excessive levels of iodine can cause autoimmune diseases and thyroid cancer. Additionally, some iodine supplements derived from kelp may contain heavy metals—supplement iodine with extreme caution. The thyroid gland influences every aspect of your health.

TESTING

Urine analysis for iodine excretion levels is very common. A blood serum analysis, however, may yield more accurate results.

Due to the characteristics of iodine and various environmental factors, I remain skeptical about the validity of iodine skin tests as an indicator of iodine deficiency. Additional testing methods are available.

HASHIMOTO'S DISEASE

As stated by the Office on Women's Health,[125] Hashimoto's disease (Hashimoto's thyroiditis) is an autoimmune disease that affects the thyroid. Thyroid hormone levels are controlled by the pituitary gland inside the brain. It makes a different hormone that triggers the production of thyroid hormone. In those suffering from Hashimoto's disease, the immune system makes antibodies that damage thyroid cells and interfere with their ability to make thyroid hormone. **Excessive iodine can trigger Hashimoto's thyroiditis** in people who are prone to getting it and occurs nearly seven times more frequently in women than men.

Over time, thyroid damage can cause thyroid hormone levels to be too low (hypothyroidism). An underactive thyroid causes every function of the body to slow down, including heart rate, brain function, and metabolism. Hashimoto's disease is the most common cause of an underactive thyroid. It is closely related to Graves' disease, another autoimmune disease that affects the thyroid.

Many people with Hashimoto's disease have no symptoms for years. An enlarged thyroid, called a *goiter*, is often the first sign of illness.

Symptoms of an underactive thyroid include:

- Fatigue
- Weight gain
- Pale, puffy face
- Feeling cold
- Joint and muscle pain
- Constipation
- Dry, thinning hair
- Heavy menstrual flow or irregular periods
- Depression
- A slowed heart rate
- Problems getting pregnant

CHAPTER SIXTEEN

POTASSIUM

Impacts: stress, heart health, bone health, cancer, insulin resistance, menopause, insomnia, infant colic, allergies, headaches, weight loss, acne, Alzheimer's, arthritis, vision, bloating, fever, gout, irritability, muscle weakness, muscular dystrophy, chronic fatigue, dermatitis

POTASSIUM WORKS AS AN ELECTROLYTE and is a critical element in maintaining a normal heartbeat rhythm. Too much or too little will result in arrhythmia (irregular heartbeat).[126] Potassium actively lowers blood pressure in people who suffer from hypertension. Hypertension dramatically increases your risk factor for cardiac arrest and stroke.[127] Growing evidence indicates low potassium intake increases the risk of atherosclerosis (hardening of the arteries) and the risk of heart attack and stroke.[128,129] However, additional studies are needed.

Individuals with physically demanding lifestyles require more potassium than those without to replenish their supply. Regularly obtaining the recommended daily adequate intake of 3,400 mg for men and 2,600 mg for women is challenging. I hope to get you over the two-thirds mark of 2,266 mg and 1,734 mg, respectively. In the end, most individuals should increase potassium intake, even if only by a few hundred milligrams each day. Moreover, reversing magnesium deficiency can significantly improve potassium utilization.

Regardless of how beneficial obtaining the recommended AI of potassium a day may be, several individuals will be able to do so for an extended period. However, establishing adequate magnesium levels significantly improves your body's utilization of potassium. It may not make up the full difference between what you consume and the recommended daily intake, but it certainly helps. In contrast, magnesium deficiency increases potassium loss via urine.[130,131]

Potassium participates in many life-giving functions, such as nerve impulse conduction, normal heart rhythm, and the regulation of blood glucose levels. It is also required to build muscle matter and burn carbohydrates for energy. Potassium is essential for every muscle contraction in your body, including cardiac, skeletal, and smooth muscle tissue.

Researchers demonstrated that individuals with higher potassium intake maintained greater bone-mineral density, thus reducing their risk of developing osteoporosis.[132]

Health issues associated with sodium often result from extremely low consumption of potassium. Potassium helps you expel sodium via your urine. Of the various supplemental forms, potassium citrate is alkaline, potassium gluconate is pH neutral, and potassium chloride is acidic. Kidneys regulate potassium levels by excreting it through the urine. Drinking excess water depletes your potassium via urination.

Potassium citrate prevents and reduces kidney stones by adhering to calcium in the urine. Potassium citrate also prevents urine from becoming too acidic.

HOW MUCH AND HOW OFTEN

As previously stated, the daily adequate intake (AI) recommendation is 3,400 mg for men and 2,600 mg for women. A typical banana contains 422 mg of potassium. Low-sodium V8, pomegranate juice, and pure coconut water are excellent sources of potassium.

Supplemental potassium can be found in tablet, capsule, salt, and powder forms. Potassium pills are regulated not to exceed 99 mg of elemental potassium. High concentrations (in pill form) can irritate or damage the stomach lining by remaining in direct contact with one area for extended periods. High doses of supplemental potassium can be harmful. I recommend not ingesting high levels of supplemental potassium unless directed to do so by a physician.

According to a five-year NHANES study comprised of 10,563 participants, the usual intake of sodium and potassium for American adults amounted to 3,569 mg/day (sodium) and 2,745 mg/day (potassium), reflecting a dietary ratio of 1.41:1. This means many adults need to consume an additional 1,880 mg of potassium a day to meet the recommended AI level. This number is even higher for individuals who drink large amounts of water or engage in high-intensity exercise. Do not supplement potassium if you have heart or kidney issues without consulting with a physician.

Supplemental potassium should always be taken with a meal to protect the stomach lining and induce a slower, more even absorption rate. If you weigh 160 pounds or more, I encourage you not to exceed 800 mg (powder or salt) in a single dose. I encourage individuals weighing less than 160 pounds not to exceed 5 mg (powder or salt) for each pound of body weight in a single dose. For example, an individual who weighs 125 pounds would not exceed 625 mg (5 mg ✕ 125) in a single dose, unless directed to do so by a physician. Again, you are encouraged not to exceed 2,400 mg of supplemental potassium in a single day, which can be accomplished in three or more separate doses with meals to mitigate stomach issues. To protect your stomach lining, you are encouraged to consult with a physician before experimenting with potassium supplements.

Admittedly, this approach may be overly cautious. When it comes to your health, a bit of caution is always warranted. Individuals with underlying health conditions such as impaired kidney function or compromised heart health should always consult with a physician before taking potassium supplements. It is possible to unknowingly suffer from impaired kidney function or some other undiagnosed condition, which may cause an otherwise safe dose of potassium to rise to dangerous levels. Supplemental potassium can be absorbed more rapidly and more completely than food-based elements. For instance, potassium in a banana is not absorbed at the same rate as supplemental potassium in a cup of water.

If you are potassium deficient, you may notice results within two days to two weeks of increased intake, including fewer muscle cramps, a more relaxed respiratory system, and more endurance during physical activities. Long-term results could include lower blood pressure, improved heart function, improved weight management, and stronger bones.

A combination of potassium-rich foods and beverages can help individuals improve their potassium levels. An informative article published in *Medical News Today* lists potassium-rich foods and their content.[133] I've added a few additional items to the list.

- Cooked or drained beet greens without salt—1,309 mg
- Canned white beans—1,189 mg
- Cooked or drained soybeans without salt—970 mg
- Cooked, boiled, or drained lima beans without salt—969 mg
- Baked sweet potato—950 mg
- 16 ounces coconut water—900 mg
- Low-sodium V8—850 mg
- Sliced avocado—708 mg
- 8 ounces pomegranate juice—600 mg
- Cooked or drained mushrooms without salt—555 mg
- Sliced banana—537 mg
- Red, ripe, raw tomatoes—427 mg
- Raw cantaloupe melon—417 mg

Table 12. Potassium—Supplement

Suggested Supplement Options	How Much and How Often
NoSalt—Potassium chloride (640 mg per 1/4 tsp)	No more than 700 mg, once or twice a day with food or large smoothie.
Morton Salt Substitute—Potassium chloride (690 mg per 1/4 tsp)	A high dosage may cause nausea.
NOW—Potassium chloride powder (365 mg per 1/8 tsp)	Consult with your physician, especially if intending to take twice per day.
NOW—Potassium citrate powder (448 mg per 1/4 tsp)	Individuals with impaired kidney function or diminished heart health should not take a potassium supplement without a doctor's approval.

ABSORPTION INHIBITORS

Alcoholic beverages and caffeine inhibit potassium absorption. More importantly, they cause your kidneys to flush additional potassium out of your system via the urine. Drinking large amounts of water will also deplete potassium due to increased urination. Low magnesium levels may increase potassium secretion from your body.

To bump up potassium levels in your diet, think about replacing one or two common food items with produce rich in potassium.

ABSORPTION ENHANCERS

Potassium is absorbed extremely well under most circumstances. Potassium needs magnesium to be fully utilized inside the body. It relies on magnesium to move across the cell membrane.[134] Therefore, reversing a magnesium deficiency greatly enhances potassium utilization.

LISTEN TO YOUR BODY

Low potassium can result in a variety of symptoms, such as muscle cramps, twitches, or weakness. It can also cause fatigue, low energy, abnormal heart rhythms, tingling or numbness sensations, confusion, depression, psychosis, delirium, and in some cases, hallucinations.

Excessive potassium levels (hyperkalemia) can be extremely hazardous. Symptoms include muscle fatigue, weakness, paralysis, abnormal heartbeat, and cardiac arrest. Individuals with healthy kidneys rarely experience issues from consuming supplemental potassium.

WARNING

When consuming adequate amounts of potassium, the human body is very efficient at managing excess via the kidneys. Nevertheless, impaired kidney function (as in diabetics) can generate dangerously high levels of potassium. It is possible for an individual to unknowingly have impaired kidney function.

TESTING

Blood serum tests for potassium levels are a poor indicator of actual tissue levels. Tissue releases its stores of various nutrients to maintain proper levels in the blood.

A sublingual epithelial cell analysis measures potassium levels within your tissue. The test kit is shipped to your local physician, who collects small, soft tissue samples from the mouth—individuals who have undergone the process state that the procedure is noninvasive and virtually painless. Tissue analysis results include levels and ratios for magnesium, phosphorus, potassium, calcium, sodium, and chloride. You are encouraged to engage in additional research before subjecting yourself to any testing procedure.

CHAPTER SEVENTEEN

CALCIUM

Impacts: bone health, heart health, nervous system, cancer

CALCIUM IS A DOUBLE-EDGED SWORD regarding heart disease. If not processed correctly, calcium can harden plaque inside the arteries. Calcium supports a wide variety of cellular activities. The body needs calcium for muscle movement, normal heart function, and to allow nerves to transmit messages between the brain and the rest of the body. Almost all calcium is stored in bones and teeth to support their structure and hardness.

As discussed in a previous chapter, the heart is largely comprised of specialized smooth muscle. When calcium flows into muscle cells, it triggers a contraction causing the heart to pump blood out. At the end of each contraction, calcium flows out of the cells, and magnesium flows in, causing muscles to relax and pull in blood. This process occurs anywhere from seventy to eighty times a minute inside an average heart when at rest.

Calcium deficiency can manifest as muscle tremors (spasms) with or without muscle cramps. It can also cause fatigue and cause an individual to feel less energetic. Low calcium levels can cause numbness or tingling sensations. Calcium deficiency has also been linked to forms of cancer.[135] Moreover, calcium deficiency can interfere with sleep and cause you to gain weight.

It is important to note that high-dosage, long-term calcium supplementation can be detrimental to your heart and increase coronary artery disease formation. Excessive calcium intake may increase incidents of heart disease and (possibly) cancer. Therefore, if an individual chooses to supplement, I suggest not exceeding 300 mg in a single dose and not to exceed 500 mg of supplemental calcium in a single day without medical supervision. Low doses, coupled with vitamin K2 supplementation, should allow your body to process calcium more effectively and minimize associated cardiovascular risks.

Adequate calcium intake is necessary for optimum health. Please consider you have likely improved calcium absorption and utilization by applying the information in previous chapters. The key is to obtain the correct amount of calcium you need and to process that calcium in a beneficial (not detrimental) way. An archived article on WebMD[136] cites Gary G. Schwartz, PhD with the following statement:

> "Many of your body's functions run on calcium, just like your laptop runs on electricity. Too little calcium in the blood can cause convulsions and too much can lead to a coma. Since your body cannot afford to oscillate between convulsions and coma, the range of serum calcium is tightly controlled."

Before your body can fully utilize calcium, you need proper vitamin D levels to absorb it. You also need a healthy liver and healthy kidneys to convert vitamin D to its active hormone. As discussed earlier, adequate magnesium and zinc levels are also essential for maximum vitamin D conversion into its active form. Once calcium is absorbed, it needs to be delivered to your bones and away from your arteries.

Vitamin K2 is the catalyst for this process.

Calcium levels in our bodies often decline as we age. As women age, their ability to absorb calcium may decrease due to reduced estrogen levels. Deficiencies in nutrients such as vitamin D, iodine, and zinc affect estrogen production. Therefore, maintaining proper levels of these critical elements serves to optimize your health in more ways than one.

HOW MUCH AND HOW OFTEN

Calcium supplements come in various forms. Calcium carbonate requires stomach acid to be absorbed and must be taken with a meal. Calcium citrate, which can be more expensive, is more readily absorbed (with or without food). Many individuals may benefit from supplementing 200–500 mg of calcium three to five days a week.

Concerns have been raised over the levels of heavy metals, such as lead and mercury, contained in coral calcium. An analysis of calcium supplements found concentrations of lead at 0.106–0.384 mg/kg in oysters, coral, and animal bone, which are considered sources of natural raw calcium. Traces of mercury and cadmium were also detected.

If you choose to supplement with coral calcium or a similar product, purchase it from a reputable manufacturer. Also, ensure the product has been tested for heavy metals and other hazardous elements, preferably by a responsible third party. The RDA for elemental calcium varies with age:

- Males and females ages nineteen to fifty (1,000 mg).
- Males ages fifty-one to seventy (1,000 mg).
- Females ages fifty-one to seventy (1,200 mg).
- Males and females age seventy-one and older (1,200 mg).

Please remember that this reflects your total calcium intake from food, drinks, and (if needed) supplements. Never supplement 50 percent or more of the RDA for calcium unless directed to do so by your physician. Furthermore, you should not take calcium supplements without also maintaining adequate (not excessive) levels of K2.

Table 13. Calcium—Food

Food Type and Quantity	How Often
Kale Broccoli Milk Yogurt Cheese Canned fish with soft bones (e.g., sardines, salmon) Orange juice (calcium fortified)	One serving of any of these items twice a day. Always consider calories and fat intake.

Table 14. Calcium—Supplement

Suggested Supplement Options	How Much and How Often
Citracal Petites—Calcium citrate (200 mg) D3 6.25 mcg (250 IU) each Pure Encapsulations—Calcium citrate (150 mg) each Bluebonnet—Calcium citrate (250 mg) D3 5 mcg (200 IU) magnesium aspartate (100 mg) each NATURELO—Plant-based calcium (150 mg) D3 (6.25 mcg) magnesium glycinate (50 mg) each	One to two pills per day, three to seven days per week. If two pills per day, consider taking them separately. Consult with your physician.

ABSORPTION INHIBITORS

Caffeine; vitamin D deficiency; magnesium deficiency; foods with phytate, such as wheat bran, pinto beans, navy beans, and peas; and foods that contain oxalates, such as beets, spinach, rhubarb, okra, tea, and sweet potatoes, inhibit calcium absorption.

ABSORPTION ENHANCERS

Vitamin D, vitamin K2, magnesium, and lysine greatly enhance the absorption and utilization of calcium. Please note that when magnesium is included in a calcium supplement, calcium will inhibit magnesium absorption.

BEST FORMULATION

- Calcium citrate (absorbs exceptionally well with food or on an empty stomach)

It would be prudent to only take one 200 mg pill at a time versus two simultaneously. Doing so may lower the risk of calcium deposit buildup inside of your arteries. Other reputable manufacturers sell high-quality calcium supplements, such as Pure Encapsulations and Bluebonnet. Choose the one that is right for you. Don't forget your K2.

LISTEN TO YOUR BODY

Calcium deficiency can present itself as fatigue, muscle cramps, muscle tremors, muscle twitches, numbness, tingling (pins and needles) sensations, impaired sleep, or having difficulty losing weight. Excess calcium may result in symptoms such as constipation or kidney stones.

WARNING

If a physician recommends supplementing more than 500 mg of calcium a day, discuss any concerns you may have regarding an increased risk of heart disease. Also, ask your physician to consider looking at your magnesium levels, vitamin K2 intake, and vitamin D levels. As a reminder, magnesium testing using epithelial cell analysis appears to be far more accurate than testing via blood analysis.

TESTING

Blood serum tests for calcium levels are very common. A sublingual epithelial cell analysis[137] may be considered for measuring calcium levels within your tissue. The test kit is shipped to your local physician, who collects small soft tissue samples from the mouth. Individuals who have undergone the process state that the procedure is noninvasive and virtually painless. You are encouraged to engage in additional research before subjecting yourself to any testing procedure.

As mentioned previously, another calcium testing method worth strong consideration is the coronary calcium scan, which looks for specks of calcium in the walls of coronary arteries.[138] There are two forms of the scan performed by two different machines—electron beam computed tomography and multidetector computed tomography. Calcifications in the coronary arteries are an early sign of coronary heart disease.[139]

CHAPTER EIGHTEEN

L-TAURINE

Impacts: estrogen, heart health, blood pressure, bone health, cancer, diabetes, osteoporosis, depression, weight loss, dementia, Alzheimer's, multiple sclerosis, autoimmune diseases, mortality, flu

AMINO ACIDS ARE MOLECULES THAT are the building blocks of proteinsTheyare primarily categorized as either essential or conditional. Essential amino acids cannot be created by the body and must be obtained via diet. Conditional amino acids can be made within the body and can also be obtained from food and supplements. Taurine is a conditional amino acid. Taurine is responsible for key functions, such as the support of electrolyte balance in the cells, maintenance of nervous system functions, the management of calcium levels in the body, and more.[140]

Taurine is one of the most plentiful amino acids in your brain, retina, muscle tissue, and organs and is given with other medications to treat congestive heart failure. It also plays a positive role in weight loss, diabetes, anxiety, and sleep disorders. Evidence indicates taurine lowers blood pressure and calms the sympathetic nervous system, reducing heart strain. Taurine also appears to provide a much deeper and sustainable sleep. As you sleep, your cardiovascular system enters an extremely beneficial state called nocturnal blood pressure dipping. More details on this critical, heart-healthy resting state will be discussed in Chapter 25 Sleep.

PREVENTING CARDIOVASCULAR DISEASE

In some cases, taurine alleviated high blood pressure. The specifics of how it manages to achieve this lies in the interactions between it and the vascular smooth muscles of blood vessels. Taurine also supports endothelial function.[141]

Additional heart-disease related research needs to be conducted on this simple amino acid. However, by preventing blood vessel problems like atherosclerosis, taurine helps maintain blood flow from the heart at a healthy pace.[142]

POSSIBLE HEARTBEAT REGULATION

While plenty of research is still ongoing, the *Journal of Dietary Supplements* noted the effects of taurine on the heart's electrical impulses.[143] Taurine interacts with potassium and the cell membranes of the heart. As discussed in the previous chapter, potassium is one of the most significant minerals needed to regulate nerve signals and muscle contractions. The presence of potassium within the heart cells allows for the proper generation of electrical impulses that cause the heart to pump life-giving blood through muscle contractions.

Taurine improves the ability of molecules to pass through the membranes (protective layer) of the cells of the heart. This process allows cells to absorb potassium more efficiently. Specifically, taurine itself is absorbed into the cells, where it then converts to an isethionic acid whose presence makes the cells more permeable.[144] Patients with heart problems like increased heart rates, irregular heartbeat, or even possible cardiac arrhythmia have noted improved functioning and reduction in palpitations when given taurine.

While categorized as a conditional amino acid, some individuals cannot produce taurine at appropriate levels, or at all. They need to obtain taurine either through their diet from taurine-rich food or supplementation. Food groups containing taurine include dairy, meat, and fish.

Incidentally, newborn babies are unable to produce taurine on their own. Their primary source is through mother's milk via breastfeeding. Some baby foods and formula also contain taurine as part of their ingredients.

Maintaining healthy levels of taurine is necessary for the proper functioning of a healthy heart.

VEGETARIANS

Taurine is primarily an animal-based amino acid. Vegetarians may be deficient in taurine. Lack of taurine associated with a meat-free diet can result in mood swings and other issues related to anxiety. Fortunately, taurine can be safely and affordably supplemented.

HOW MUCH AND HOW OFTEN

Taurine appears to be safe at high levels. Good results seem to occur within a daily intake range of 1,000 to 2,500 mg. Here is where supplement abuse often begins. Individuals sometimes forget to consider that some, if not all, of their daily requirements are either obtained by the food they eat or created within them. They decide to supplement 100 percent (or more) of their need, which, in many cases, is unnecessary. There is no RDA for taurine at this time.

One study gave participants 9,000 mg per day for one year without side effects. However, reports also indicate there is little to no added benefit by exceeding 3,500 mg per day. Please keep in mind that many individuals obtain taurine via food. Also, taurine is produced naturally in the body.

If you decide to take supplemental taurine, I suggest not exceeding 2,000 mg per day unless directed to do so by your physician. Some bloggers are overselling taurine with claims that have yet to be thoroughly vetted. Many individuals consume higher doses of this supplement than I recommend without any reported side effects. However, overuse of taurine supplements on an empty stomach can result in acid reflux, resulting from increased stomach acid secretion. Taking it with a meal may reduce this risk but may also diminish absorption.

If you are taurine deficient, you may notice results within two days to two weeks. Short-term results may include deeper sleep (especially when taken with magnesium) and an increased frequency of memorable dreams. Long-term results may include improved heart function. Search *taurine benefits* online, and you will be amazed at the findings.

Table 15. L-Taurine—Food

Food Type and Quantity	How Often
Whole capelin (6,174 mg) Cooked Dungeness crab (5,964 mg) Alaskan salmon fillets (4,401 mg) Lamb (3,676 mg)	One serving of any of these items once a day. Always consider calories and fat intake.

Table 16. L-Taurine—Supplement

Suggested Supplement Options	How Much and How Often
Solgar—Taurine (500 mg) Jarrow Formulas—Taurine Pharmaceutical Grade (1,000 mg)	500–1,500 mg four to six days per week with food. Or a combination of foods (listed above) and supplements. Take with 133 to 200 mg of chelated magnesium with dinner for a deeper sleep.

ABSORPTION INHIBITORS

Albeit there does not appear to be any direct inhibitors of taurine absorption, food, in general, appears to retard taurine absorption to some degree.

ABSORPTION ENHANCERS

Taurine is best absorbed on an empty stomach or following an intense workout. However, this increases the possibility of developing ulcers. Your body's natural taurine production is enhanced by vitamin A, vitamin D3 25 mcg (1,000 IU), P5P, and zinc.

BEST FORMULATION

Both Jarrow Formulas (1,000 mg) and Solgar (500 mg) taurine come in capsule form. GNC sells taurine in pill form. Any reputable manufacturer may be considered.

PERSONAL

Just 500 mg of taurine made me a little sluggish for a couple of hours. I have since ceased taking taurine during the day. Taking 500 mg of taurine three to five nights per week after dinner, coupled with 200 mg of magnesium (with dinner), resulted in a much deeper sleep. It also led to more frequent, vivid, memorable dreams that seem to continue for longer durations.

WARNING

There is one report of brain damage in a bodybuilder who took nearly 14 grams of taurine (14,000 mg) along with insulin and steroids. It is not known which of the substances or combination of substances, if any, caused the injury.

High doses of taurine can increase stomach acid levels, which can result in heartburn and peptic ulcers. In addition, a product reviewer stated having a noticeable impairment to their short-term memory after taking taurine. The reviewer went on to state that their short-term memory returned to normal after ceasing taurine supplementation.

TESTING

Measuring taurine levels in whole blood appears to yield more accurate results than measuring levels contained within blood plasma.

CHAPTER NINETEEN

LIVER HEALTH

ANOTHER TOPIC RARELY DISCUSSED IS the liver's role in heart health. Every minute, a healthy liver will filter more than two quarts of blood pumped from the heart. The liver also produces a much-needed substance called bile to remove fat from inside the blood vessels.[145] Research indicates a compromised liver contributes to the development of **atherosclerosis** (hardening of the arteries).[146] Unfortunately, many liver diseases, such as nonalcoholic fatty liver disease (NAFLD), often go undiagnosed. NAFLD symptoms include fatigue or pain in the abdomen's upper right side where your liver is located.

In 2018, Poland's Department of Infectious Diseases and Hepatology found significant associations between NAFLD and various heart conditions. [147]

> "The incidences of coronary artery calcification, hypertension, aortic valve sclerosis, diastolic dysfunction, atherosclerotic plaques, and increased carotid intima-media thickness were more common in patients with NAFLD than in those without."
> —**Department of Infectious Diseases and Hepatology**

Many of your body's nutrients are stored in the liver, such as vitamins A, D, E, and K. Overwhelming your liver with excessive amounts of any substance will not make it perform better. Everything in the human body has a breakover threshold, meaning adding more of substance X will yield diminishing returns and can eventually be harmful. Diminished liver function adversely impacts vitamin D levels and the production of other important hormones, such as osteoprotegerin. In turn, reduced levels of these hormones drastically impede the formation of dense, healthy bone.

Alcohol abuse can cause cirrhosis of the liver, thereby diminishing your liver's function. Constant intake of processed food and poorly prepared fatty meals can result in a fatty, poorly functioning liver. No one will ever achieve a perfect diet. The goal here is to be mindful of how important your liver is to your cardiovascular system, life expectancy, and overall health.

A ten-year study published in *Hepatology* shows liver injury caused by herbals and dietary supplements (HDS) has increased from 7 percent to 20 percent. High doses of green tea extract (camellia sinensis) have been identified as a significant cause of liver injury.[148] Many retailers boast of having high concentrations of this ingredient in their products to burn fat. A searchable database produced by the National Institute of Diabetes and Digestive and Kidney Diseases (NIDDK) identifying harmful products can be found at a website called *LiverTox*. A report in the database reports a patient developed nausea, abdominal pain and jaundice four months after starting a weight loss supplement. Green tea extract was the predominant ingredient of the supplement.[149]

- https://livertox.nih.gov/ (URL is subject to change)

DRUG-INDUCED LIVER INJURY NETWORK (DILIN)

The NIDDK established the DILIN to evaluate the impact of medications and dietary supplements on the liver. The main results of their investigation are cited below. [150]

> "Liver injury due to herbal and dietary supplements (HDS) increased from 7 percent to 20 percent during the study period. Bodybuilding HDS caused prolonged jaundice (median 91 days) in young men but did not result in any fatalities or liver transplantation. The remaining HDS cases presented as hepatocellular injury, predominantly in middle-aged women and more frequently led to death or transplantation compared to injury from medications."

More information about the DILIN is available at their website:

- https://dilin.org/

CENTER FOR DRUG EVALUATION AND RESEARCH (CDER)

According to its website, the Food and Drug Administration's (FDA) Center for Drug Evaluation and Research (CDER) promotes and protects the health of Americans by ensuring that all prescription and over-the-counter drugs are safe and effective. The CDER serves as a consumer watchdog for the more than ten thousand drugs on the market.

The CDER routinely monitors TV, radio, and print drug ads to ensure they are truthful and balanced. They also play a critical role in providing health professionals and consumers with information, enabling them to use drugs appropriately and safely. Please visit CDER for a current list of tainted supplements at:

- https://tinyurl.com/mg232tg

According to the CDER, the list of 1,051 tainted products in their database as of January 12, 2021, reflects only a small fraction of the potentially hazardous products marketed to consumers. Even if a product is not included in this list, consumers should exercise caution before using certain products.

PAMPER YOUR LIVER

One approach to protect your liver (besides ending bad habits) is to drink a glass of *lemon water* from time to time—perhaps once per week. Some suggest doing so more frequently.

Cut a fresh lemon, add a few slices into a glass of room-temperature water (squeeze the juice into the water first), and allow it to sit for several minutes, then enjoy! Please note that the acidic nature of lemons can erode tooth enamel over time. It is recommended that you use a straw, rinse after drinking, or brush your teeth when done.

Besides lemon water, there are several foods and beverages available to you that can pamper your liver. The list includes milk thistle, green tea (not extract), grapefruit (and juice), beets (and juice), broccoli, brussels sprouts, mustard greens, walnuts, fatty fish (not fried), blueberries, and cranberries (including juice). Add a few—or all—these items to your menu as often as you like. A byproduct of eating healthier is better weight management and more sustained energy.

Also, organic produce has been shown to decrease the level of chemical toxins in individuals. However, organic food is often far more expensive than other produce. Unfortunately, some people cannot afford it. Nevertheless, you are encouraged to add some or all of the products previously listed to your diet, even if you opt for nonorganic varieties.

Heart health is not an all-or-nothing process. Any improvements you can reasonably accomplish for your liver will help your cardiovascular system and overall health. Simply do what you can.

CHAPTER TWENTY

OBESITY

OBESITY RATES HAVE SKYROCKETED WITHIN the USA and the world at large. If this trend continues, average life expectancy could decrease despite medical advances. Being overweight or obese dramatically increases your risk of developing numerous adverse health conditions. According to the CDC, in 1990, ten states had a prevalence of obesity less than 10 percent, and no state had a prevalence equal to or greater than 15 percent.[151]

By 2010, no state had a prevalence of obesity less than 20 percent. Thirty-six states had a prevalence equal to or greater than 25 percent; twelve of these states had a prevalence equal to or greater than 30 percent. According to the National Health and Nutrition Examination Survey, 2013–2014:[152,153,154,155,156]

36 percent of White adults were defined as obese, and just under 8 percent deemed to have extreme obesity.

48 percent of Black adults were defined as obese, and just over 12 percent deemed to have extreme obesity.

42.6 percent of Hispanic adults were found to be obese, and just over 7 percent were deemed to have extreme obesity.

Only 12.6 percent of Asian adults were considered obese.

Figure 5. 2019 Obesity Rates in US Adults by State [157]

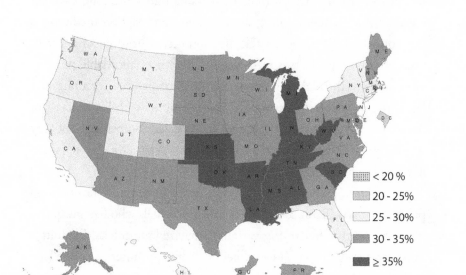

Unfortunately, a segment of society has chosen to turn a blind eye toward this health crisis. Glamorizing obesity encourages people to view it as something to aspire to versus a deadly condition to avoid. Individuals who speak out publicly against this epidemic are accused of fat-shaming and are vilified on social media. The scientific community has grown eerily silent on this topic.

Obesity kills nearly three million people a year globally and 300,000 people a year in the United States alone. Consequently, anyone concerned about the death toll of COVID-19 should be even more concerned by the growing death toll of obesity. Obesity was a primary cofactor in several deaths and hospitalizations attributed to COVID-19, especially in economically challenged communities. Moreover, obesity is a major cofactor in other fatal diseases, such as cancer. Many wonderful individuals are struggling with this challenging condition. Obesity is a rapidly growing, deadly epidemic that can no longer be ignored.

For some, obesity is entirely by choice. Others, however, desperately seek solutions. Unfortunately, fad diets, gimmicky machines, and harmful weight-loss products transformed desperation into a multibillion-dollar industry. Age, genetics, eating disorders, and prescription medications can contribute to obesity. Lack of resources, education, and health care are also major factors to overcome. The most affordable produce often contains the highest levels of pesticides, empty calories, unhealthy fat, and **genetic modifications** (GMO), coupled with lower levels of micronutrients needed to fuel metabolic processes. Surprisingly, obesity is also a growing issue in the ranks of fame and wealth, which is apparent in the entertainment industry.

Considering the litany of faux diets and harmful fat-burning products, it is difficult to simply blame individuals who feel incapable of losing weight after trying various publicized gimmicks. Exploitive infomercials and magic gadgets filled with false promises can often lead to despair. Nevertheless, real long-term solutions do exist.

GOOD NEWS

Readily available micronutrients can play an integral role in combating obesity. Yet, they are often overlooked. Rarely is an individual struggling with their weight asked, "Are you getting enough zinc? How about magnesium?" These and other nutrients play a critical role in metabolic processes. To be clear, reversing nutrient deficiencies alone is not a cure for obesity. However, it is a highly effective strategy to greatly enhance one's effort to achieve and maintain a healthy weight.

For many, obesity can be prevented and even reversed. Doing so requires accurate knowledge, realistic expectations, commitment, and resources. Proper nutrition, physical activity, stress management, mood, and weight monitoring are all proven to prevent and reverse excessive weight gain. When you take steps to prevent weight gain or lose excessive weight, you also lower your risk of developing heart disease, diabetes, stroke, and other health issues. Here are some highly effective weapons to repel and defeat obesity.

FIBER

Dietary fiber is highly underrated by most individuals. It significantly enhances weight loss and lowers LDL (bad) cholesterol. Moreover, fiber is among the most accessible and affordable substances to obtain, yet few individuals consume adequate levels. One of the best actions anyone can take to maintain a healthy weight or lose weight is to regularly consume food containing high levels of fiber.

Foods that are high in fiber include peas, lentils, beans, barley, acorn squash, raspberries, blackberries, and seeds. Daily, women should obtain 25 grams of fiber and men should obtain 28 grams.

I lost twenty-four pounds by switching from coffee to green tea, limiting alcoholic beverages, increasing fiber intake, reducing stress, and reversing micronutrient deficiencies. I use salad plates instead of dinner plates to control meal portions. At six feet and one inch, 202 pounds, I am in a far more comfortable place than my peak weight of 226 pounds.

Every other day, I make a meal-replacement smoothie packed with fiber from blueberries, blackberries, raspberries, and a bit of shredded coconut to avoid gaining weight. I add one half serving of Optimum Nutrition's whey-isolate protein powder, and I sometimes add a tablespoon of acacia powder. The mixed berries I use are nothing special, just a premixed selection located in the frozen-fruit section of most grocery stores. I also add an organic banana and frozen strawberries. Kale and avocado are additional options to consider. I eat a bowl of *original* Fiber-One cereal every other day, if not every day, with or without adding cinnamon and honey.

I prefer 100 percent grass-fed, organic, 2 percent milk fat, which can be pricey. Any 2 percent milk that fits your budget will do. Some view cow's milk as unhealthy. I drink organic, grass-fed cow's milk every day. Rather than blame the cow, from which humans have been drinking for millennia, I hold today's farmers responsible for what they put in the cow, such as genetically modified animal grain feed, corn, pesticides, and artificial hormones (or chemical hormone enhancers). I hold them accountable by not buying their tainted products.

Unfortunately, too many individuals seeking healthy alternatives cannot afford this *luxury*. Initially, healthier food choices indeed are often more expensive. However, in the long run, healthy food options are not as expensive as they appear due to fewer medical expenses, fewer prescription drugs, and often higher earning potential resulting from nutrition-enhanced focus, energy, and cognitive abilities. Healthier food choices offer an excellent return on investment.

Additional sources of fiber include mashed cauliflower, and broccoli. Having a bowl of Fiber-One cereal a few times per week will help to peel the pounds away. Apples and pears are also tasty fiber treats. Naturally occurring sugars are not the issue that some individuals make them out to be when consumed in moderation. The benefits for weight management offered by fruit and some whole grains outweigh the impact of the sugars they contain. Sugar derived from doughnuts, cotton candy, and potato chips is an entirely different story.

Develop the habit of reading food nutrition labels for fiber content. It is easier to focus more on the recommended dietary allowance percentage versus the grams. It is also important to take magnesium supplements, not just for the myriad of health benefits but also to soften your fiber-enriched stool. Magnesium is also very beneficial for weight management.

If frozen meals are a part of your diet, consider brands such as Evol and Healthy Choice. Healthy Choice Mediterranean Lentil Steamers are packed with fiber and micronutrients. Also, opt for Veggie Lasagna over Meat Lovers. This suggestion is for those who include frozen meals as a regular part of their diet. I am by no means suggesting anyone should view frozen dinners as the best dietary option.

However, any change you are willing to make and sustain is better than no change at all. Regardless of your lifestyle, obtaining adequate (not excessive) levels of fiber and key nutrients is extremely beneficial to weight loss and weight management. It is often the missing link to a healthier weight.

The following nutrients directly impact weight management:

- Magnesium lowers the level of fasting glucose and insulin. Moreover, magnesium greatly enhances the body's ability to utilize potassium. Magnesium is essential for multiple weight management, energy, and metabolic functions. Magnesium deficiency is a global issue, which can quickly be reversed.
- Potassium helps build muscle and burn carbohydrates for energy. Most Americans fall far short of the recommended daily intake. Improving potassium levels and reversing magnesium deficiency increases the body's ability to burn carbs.
- Zinc is incredibly beneficial for metabolism. Obese individuals typically present significantly lower than normal zinc levels. Zinc is also critical to testosterone production, which also supports weight management.
- Vitamin D enhances weight loss and weight management. A large segment of the population is vitamin D deficient.
- Taurine burns fat, slows weight gain, and promotes weight loss. It also appears to aid in achieving higher quality sleep, which is critical for weight management.
- Iodine directly supports thyroid health. The thyroid greatly influences an array of metabolic functions and energy levels. Today, the thyroid is bombarded by chemicals, such as bromide, fluoride, and chloride that it mistakes for iodide. Therefore, it is imperative to maintain adequate (not excessive) iodine intake.

There is much more to discuss about this topic, including the high concentrations of hormone influencing toxins associated with fast-food consumption.[158,159] However, the information provided can genuinely help with taking control of your weight. Please refer to the associated chapters for more details on the micronutrients listed here.

Achieving a healthier weight is a significant triumph for deterring cardiovascular disease. Individuals do not gain weight overnight. Therefore, they should not attempt to lose it too rapidly. Weight management is a marathon, not a sprint.

CHAPTER TWENTY-ONE

CARBOHYDRATES AND PROTEIN

Impacts: energy, weight loss, bone health, heart health, brain health

HEALTHY CARBOHYDRATES ARE THE BODY'S primary fuel source for physical endurance, brain activity, and internal processes to maintain a strong heart. Not all carbs are created equal. Carbohydrates derived from beans, chickpeas, and wild rice have a much healthier impact than cookies, doughnuts, pound cake, and soda.

Healthy carbohydrates provide several important micronutrients and allow for the stable release of glucose for adenosine triphosphate (ATP) energy. In addition, some forms of healthy carbs are high in fiber, which is critical for sustaining a more even rate of food absorption and weight management. Contrary to misinformation from faux diets, healthy carbs can be very beneficial to weight management, focus, and energy.

Exercise is integral to heart health and the prevention of cardiovascular disease. Reduced fatigue and improved exercise performance have been associated with multiple transportable carbohydrates rather than a single carbohydrate.[160] Healthy, carbohydrate-rich foods provide a readily available source of fuel for muscle glycogen synthesis. Glycogen synthesis restores energy reserves in the liver and skeletal muscle.

Moreover, a well-kept secret is chronically low potassium intake is a major contributor to the difficulty of metabolizing carbohydrates. Low potassium adversely impacts many vital functions, such as heart rhythm and insulin resistance.

Here again, diet-fad enthusiasts view carbohydrates as a problem to eliminate. The inability to burn carbohydrates may be a symptom of a far more detrimental health issue or a nutrient deficiency. Excessive simple carbohydrate consumption can be harmful to your health. However, a balanced intake of healthy carbohydrates is highly beneficial.

HEALTHY CARBOHYDRATE OPTIONS

- Sweet potatoes
- Blueberries
- Legumes
- High fiber oatmeal
- Acorn squash
- Barley
- Buckwheat
- Cauliflower
- Brown rice
- Quinoa

In a pinch, your body will burn fat for fuel. When fat stores are depleted, your body will burn protein to survive. Make no mistake, your cells and your brain prefer complex carbohydrates as their primary source of fuel. A moderately active person should consume approximately 275 grams of healthy carbohydrates a day.

PROTEIN

Protein is one of the body's most utilized sources for skeletal muscle, soft tissue, and brain function. Inadequate protein intake is extremely unhealthy and can lead to growth retardation (in children), muscle-mass reduction, poor bone structure, decreased immunity, and heart disease. Older men who exhibit protein deficiency have higher incidents of osteoporotic fracture.[161,162] The heart is a specialized muscle. Adequate protein intake is necessary for a sound and healthy heart.

However, excessive protein can cause harmful conditions in individuals with impaired liver or kidney function. Excessive protein, coupled with low mineral intake, can lower serum pH, resulting in acidosis. Severe acidosis can adversely impact heart strength and function. You can counteract the acidic effects of excess protein with fruits and dark green vegetables. Also, ensure you obtain adequate (not excessive) magnesium, potassium, and calcium to maintain nutrient balance. Consuming more protein than you need will not force your body to use the excess. Anything your body cannot store or process becomes waste. Balance is key.

Processed meat ranks among the unhealthiest sources of protein. In contrast, salmon and tuna are among the most beneficial sources because of their higher omega-3 fatty acids content. One must be careful with farm-raised salmon as it may contain unhealthy levels of mercury when consumed frequently. Wild-caught salmon is safer. Unfortunately, it is also more expensive.

Weight-based protein calculators:

- https://www.calculatorpro.com/calculator/protein-calculator
- https://www.bodybuilding.com/fun/calpro.htm

VEGETARIANS

Vegetarians can get enough basic protein via plants. However, important amino acids, such as L-taurine and L-lysine, are only abundant in animal-based protein. L-lysine is one of nine essential amino acids that cannot be manufactured by your body. Fortunately, L-taurine and L-lysine can be supplemented.

HOW MUCH AND HOW OFTEN

Recent data suggests overall daily protein intake for a moderately active person should fall between 0.4 g and 0.8 g of protein per pound of bodyweight. Those undertaking advanced exercise regimens require higher protein intake, possibly in the range of 0.8 to 1.3 g per pound of bodyweight. These are just ballpark figures. Professional athlete requirements are even higher.

Beverages such as milk contain protein and carbohydrates. When using protein powders with milk or juice, add the number of grams (g) listed on the milk or juice label with the amount contained in the powder to determine the total intake.

Table 17. Protein—Food

Food Type and Quantity	How Often
Tuna, chicken, turkey, bison, lean beef or pork, wild salmon, tilapia, whitefish, cage-free eggs, milk, cheese (dairy), beans, seeds, nuts, nut butter	One serving of any of these items two or three times a day.

Table 18. Protein—Supplement

Suggested Supplement Options	How Much and How Often
Optimum Nutrition—Whey Protein Isolate Powder (or any reputable manufacturer) Blackberries, blueberries, and acacia powder are excellent sources of fiber to include with your protein. Mixing with organic milk provides additional calcium.	0.1 to 0.2 grams per pound of body weight every other day or as needed. 0.15 to 0.25 grams per pound of bodyweight for advanced exercise regimens. Supplemental protein should NOT provide the bulk of your daily requirement.

ABSORPTION INHIBITORS

Protein absorption is rarely inhibited within a healthy GI tract.

ABSORPTION ENHANCERS

Papaya, cheeses, and certain vegetables provide digestive enzymes to more effectively break down protein-rich meals.

BEST FORMULATION

- Whey isolate protein powder (absorbs exceptionally well)
- Optimum Nutrition's Whey Protein Powder contains 24 g of protein, 5.5 g of branched-chain amino acids (BCAAs), and 4 g of glutamine per serving. It is loaded with whey protein isolates.

LISTEN TO YOUR BODY

Protein deficiency symptoms include skin discoloration, skin rashes, lethargy, fatigue, difficulty sleeping, excessive sleeping (lack of energy), muscle weakness, muscle loss, frequent infections, slow wound healing, hair loss, brittle hair, mood swings, depression, anxiety, and apathy. Excessive protein may present itself as low calcium, gout, or kidney stones.

WARNING

Excessive protein intake may trigger your body to release calcium from your bones. Also, there are some health risks associated with excessive protein intake for individuals with impaired kidney or liver function. Additional risks may be present because of cancer-promoting agents found in some protein sources or introduced by food preparation.

CHAPTER TWENTY-TWO

MULTIVITAMINS AND MINERALS

MULTIVITAMINS AND MINERALS (MVM) ARE compilations of vitamins, minerals, and trace elements needed to sustain physical and mental well-being. A quality MVM will provide additional nutrient requirements for optimal heart health, such as folate (folic acid).

According to the National Institutes of Health, "Several studies have found that MVM users tend to have higher micronutrient intakes from their diet than nonusers. Ironically, the populations at highest risk of nutritional inadequacy who might benefit the most from MVMs are the least likely to take them."[163]

An editorial published by the *Annals of Internal Medicine* claimed that vitamin and mineral supplements are a waste of money.[164] I could not disagree more. Upon reading the article, certain statements caught my attention, such as:

> "Efficacy of vitamin supplements for primary prevention in community-dwelling adults with no nutritional deficiencies."

"Use of a multivitamin supplement in a well-nourished elderly population did not prevent cognitive decline."

I agree with the conclusion that vitamin and mineral supplements may not benefit people who are *well-nourished* and people "with no nutritional deficiencies." If you are nutritionally whole, you will not gain added benefits from multivitamins. The poorly considered editorial resulted in the following headlines:

"Experts: Don't Waste Your Money on Multivitamins." (*WebMD*)

"Vitamins Lack Clear Health Benefits, May Pose Risks." (*Forbes*)

"Medical journal: 'Case closed' against vitamin pills." (*USA Today*)

The message conveyed by these and other news articles is very troubling. They may persuade individuals suffering from nutritional deficiencies to avoid supplements that can improve their health. Individuals living with nutrient deficiencies can benefit immensely from quality supplementation. The very purpose of supplements is to fill in the areas where individuals are not nutritionally whole.

The Harvard School of Public Health states, "Looking at all the evidence, the potential health benefits of taking a standard daily multivitamin seem to outweigh the potential risks for most people."[165] Furthermore, The Agency for Healthcare Research and Quality states, "Multivitamin/mineral supplement use may prevent cancer in individuals with poor or suboptimal nutritional status."[166]

Specialized formulations of MVMs are recommended and sometimes prescribed for prenatal care. This is likely because a high-quality MVM is far more efficient at filling a broad spectrum of nutritional gaps. They cannot and should not be used in place of healthy food choices. They most definitely should be used to *top off* your nutritional tank when diet alone does not meet all your nutrient requirements. I have personally witnessed the impact of a high-quality MVM on several individuals. All MVMs are not equal; quality matters.

HOW MUCH AND HOW OFTEN

Try any high-quality MVM six days a week for up to thirty days, either in half doses or at full strength. If you do not notice any results, many retailers offer full refunds. A comprehensive list of several MVM products to choose from can be found at www.MultivitaminGuide.org.

Quite often, a high-quality MVM will turn your urine into a vibrant yellowish hue. Don't panic. This is mainly the excess B-12 flushing out of your system. If you are nutrient deficient, your energy and mental focus should noticeably increase within a few days or a few weeks. The more nutrient deficient you are, the quicker and more noticeable the results should be. If you are prone to coughs, illness, or infections, you may experience a decrease in frequency, severity, and duration. There are many benefits that a high-quality MVM can offer individuals with mild to severe nutrient deficiencies.

High-quality MVMs cost much more than the more familiar brands. As with most things, you get what you pay for. I assign a four-tier categorization based on overall quality to MVMs. The fourth tier is the worst, and the first tier is the best. Each tier consists of several brands. Fortunately, over the years, first-tier brand prices have dramatically decreased. They initially sold for as much as $120 for a one-month supply. They currently sell for about half of what they once did, which is still somewhat expensive for the average household. However, first-tier MVM products require fewer additional supplements.

I usually recommend the second-tier range, which costs around $18 for a one-month supply. However, you may need to augment them with two or three additional standalone supplements, which drives up the cost. A monthly price breakdown for recommended MVMs is contained in Chapter 24 under *Product List*. Prices are subject to change.

First-tier and second-tier brands have an exceedingly high absorption rate. Consider taking only one-half or less of the recommended dose. If the manufacturer's recommendation is two or three pills a day, only take one. If you are meticulous, you can break one tablet in half to take one part with breakfast and the other portion during lunch. Individuals who drink alcohol excessively or maintain a poor diet may require the full recommended dose. I recommend skipping two or three days a week to excrete excess nutrients accrued through MVMs and diet. One can either skip consecutive days or alternating days based on one's lifestyle.

First-tier MVMs frequently contain an exceptionally balanced ratio of vitamins, minerals, and trace elements. Second-tier MVMs are typically less balanced and contain fewer micronutrients. Third and fourth tier MVMs are of extremely poor quality and may sell for as low as $25 for a one-year supply (approx. $2.08 per month). They use the least desirable forms of vitamins and minerals and are one step removed from a placebo. They seem to put more money into TV advertisements than the vitamins themselves. In the long run, high-quality MVMs are also more cost-effective due to health benefits.

Many second-tier MVMs, and below, contain one or two low-quality mineral formulations, such as magnesium oxide. As previously stated, low-quality mineral formulations do not absorb well. Additionally, minerals compete for the same absorption receptors, causing some minerals to inhibit others' absorption.

Excess nutrients from MVMs combined with a nutrient-dense diet can introduce health problems. Individuals who regularly take MVMs typically maintain a healthier diet than those who do not. If your diet is reasonably sound, moderate your MVM intake. You simply do not need as much as individuals with low-nutrition diets.

You may only need a half dose (or less) of MVM three or four days per week. There is no benefit from overdosing nutrients except correcting a deficiency or offsetting unique health conditions. Doing so merely wastes money and can be detrimental to your long-term health. If your diet is nutrient poor, taking the full recommended serving five to seven days may be required initially, but not forever.

Table 19. Multivitamins Ratings (MultivaminGuide.org—Top 10 of 100)[167]

Company	Product
NATURELO Premium Supplements	Whole Food Multivitamin
Xtend-Life Natural Products	Total Balance
Douglas Laboratories	Ultra Preventive X
USANA Health Sciences	HealthPak
Dr. Mercola	Whole Food Multivitamin PLUS
Shaklee	Vitalizer
Life Extension	Life Extension Mix
Metagenics	Wellness Essentials
Nutrilite (Amway)	Double X
Garden of Life	Vitamin Code

View the current list at http://www.multivitaminguide.org

ABSORPTION INHIBITORS

Absorption can be inhibited by phytate and caffeine.

ABSORPTION ENHANCERS

Multivitamins/minerals are absorbed best when taken with a meal.

BEST FORMULATION

- Xtend-Life Natural Products—Total Balance
- Douglas Laboratories—Ultra Preventive X
- NATURELO—Whole Food Multivitamin
- Life Extension—Life Extension Mix
- Life Extension—Two-Per-Day (capsule or tablet)
- Optimum Nutrition—Opti-Men/Opti-Women

If you are currently taking an MVM found at your typical drugstore, you are encouraged to switch to a higher-quality brand. MVMs found in most drugstores seemingly spend massive amounts of money on commercials as opposed to better ingredients. This benefits their bottom line but does very little for your short- and long-term health. It is often true that something is better than nothing. However, investing in better-quality MVMs can yield much more significant results when it comes to your health.

Purchase MVMs from a reputable vitamin store or directly from the manufacturer's website. Third-party websites that do not specialize in health and nutrition have spotty quality control. Some individuals have received counterfeit or expired products.

LISTEN TO YOUR BODY

General symptoms of a deficiency may include fatigue, insomnia, hair loss, dry skin, headache, depression, anxiety, frequent infections, and slow healing. Excess consumption may cause stomach cramps, nausea, or diarrhea.

WARNING

Multivitamins can irritate your stomach, especially if not taken with a meal. Quality multivitamins contain high concentrations of nutrients. You likely only need one half or less of the manufacturer's suggested dose. I also encourage skipping a day (or two) each week to purge excess from your system.

CHAPTER TWENTY-THREE

SUPPLEMENT ABUSE

ACCORDING TO *MERRIAM-WEBSTER,* **A SUPPLEMENT** is "something that is added to something else in order to make it complete." [168] Unfortunately, some people have convinced themselves and others that their bodies function better with excessive supplementation instead of a balanced ratio. Moreover, some commercialized doctors who profit from the vitamin industry perpetuate the need for massive doses of supplements to pad their wallets.

As discussed previously, iodine supplement abuse recently ignited into an online fad. Although the RDA for iodine is only 150 mcg (micrograms) per day, individuals have suggested daily supplementation as high as 12.5 mg (milligrams) a day. This is more than eighty-three times the RDA. As previously stated, the belief that people in Japan consume 13.8 mg of iodine a day may have resulted from an incorrectly applied equation used in a research paper written in 1967.

As of 2004, the average iodine intake in the United States ranged from 138 to 353 mcg (micrograms) per day. [169] Based on these actual intake levels, if 12.5 mg (milligrams) of daily iodine were required to maintain thyroid health (as suggested by mega-dosers), one would expect most of the US population to develop goiter and other dramatic health issues associated with severe iodine deficiency. Also, early-stage brain development would be severely impaired in newborns. Implying that people are severely iodine deficient without displaying known, associated symptoms is very problematic, to say the least, and extremely misleading. However, it is possible that we need to consume a little more iodine than the RDA due to environmental factors, such as elevated fluoride and bromide intake in industrialized countries.

Moreover, how much you consume of any nutrient is not indicative of how much you absorb. For instance, your body will absorb far more magnesium from 200 mg of chelated magnesium glycinate than it will from 200 mg of magnesium oxide. Mega-dosers often fail to account for varying absorption rates between different formulations.

Individuals who mega-dose without medical supervision:

- May not have their kidneys or liver periodically tested for stress or damage
- Will likely mega-dose on multiple supplements
- May base their decision to mega-dose on one-off studies, speculation, misinformation, or current fads
- May not be aware that articles supporting mega-dosing on a supplement often rely on very few sources versus a preponderance of credible, independent research
- Ignore the compilation of scientific studies conducted in multiple countries that draw similar conclusions regarding adequate levels required for health
- Appear to ignore the amount of nutrients they are naturally obtaining from food and beverages

BALANCE WORKS BETTER

When used properly, supplements can be very effective at maintaining one's health and performance. In general, people who take supplements make healthier food choices. Hence, individuals with healthier diets require lower doses of supplemental nutrients than those who maintain a less healthy diet. Mega-dosing on supplements can undermine one's investment in healthy lifestyle choices.

The human body is an extremely complex biological machine. Nutrients are like the fuel-air-spark mixture in your car's engine whereby too much or too little of any one ingredient will make your engine run poorly, create more toxins, produce less energy, and shorten its life. Cells require the right amount of oxygen, fluids, vitamins, minerals, and micronutrients to operate at their peak. Overwhelming them with supplements may give you a short-term boost, but unfortunately, it may also diminish other vital functions and even shorten your life.

I am a strong advocate for filling nutritional holes via supplementation. I stand *firmly against* those who encourage abusing supplements to achieve a singular result.

CHAPTER TWENTY-FOUR

DAILY SUPPLEMENT SCHEDULES

DAILY SUPPLEMENT SCHEDULES HAVE BEEN developed according to the typical income, lifestyle, and nutritional needs of specific age groups. Proceed with caution, especially if you are taking medications, have allergies, or have an underlying health condition. Also, consider consulting with your doctor before adopting a schedule.

Potassium, protein, and carbohydrates have not been added to the schedules. Please refer to the *How Much and How Often* section of their associated chapters for more details. Additionally, please refer to Chapter 19 Liver Health for a list of foods that promote liver health.

You will also find that taurine is not included in the daily schedules. Although taurine demonstrates a positive role in weight loss, diabetes, anxiety, and sleep disorders, more studies are needed. If you elect to take supplemental taurine, consider taking 500–1500 mg, four to six days per week. High concentrations on an empty stomach can increase stomach acid secretion, potentially resulting in acid reflux.

Due to many variables and factors, you may need to deviate from the schedules provided to address unique conditions. For example, the more direct sun exposure you obtain—based on your region and lifestyle—the less vitamin D supplementation you require.

MULTIVITAMINS AND MINERALS (MVM)

The Life Extension Two-Per-Day MVM is the example used in the following schedules. The manufacturer's suggested dosage is two tablets per day with meals. However, only one tablet per day is recommended in the schedules.

Each schedule suggests that you only take half (or less) of the manufacturer's suggested dose for several reasons. These are high-quality multivitamins for the cost, which means they contain formulations of nutrients that will be readily absorbed into your system, so much so that your urine may turn bright yellow or orange. Do not let this discoloration alarm you, as it is merely your kidneys disposing of excess vitamin B-12.

When you purchase better-quality MVMs, you typically need less than 50 percent of the manufacturer's recommended usage. You can take fewer capsules or break a tablet in half to accomplish this. Moreover, you may only need to take it three to five days per week. Additionally, you will receive nutrients from food, beverages, and other standalone vitamin products. The goal is to achieve balance. You are encouraged to go one or more days per week without taking a MVM to allow your body time to metabolize or purge excess.

There are MVM products available of even higher quality. However, they are more cost-prohibitive, as indicated in the product list following the *Daily Supplement Schedules*. If you choose to move up to the more expensive brands, you will need fewer additional standalone products to fill in the gaps. This increases convenience and offsets some of the added costs.

IMPORTANT: You can take multivitamins with breakfast or lunch. I caution against taking them with your last meal because it could result in bouts of insomnia.

THE TOTAL APPROACH

When taking supplements, you should always consider the total nutrient intake and likely absorption rate. For example, Life Extension

Two-Per-Day contains 25 mcg (1,000 IU) of vitamin D3 in each pill. Citracal Petites contain 6.25 mcg (250 IU) of vitamin D3 in each tablet. A glass of milk also has vitamin D.

When you combine the total amount of vitamin D provided from all sources, how much more do you require from a standalone supplement, if any? It is also advisable to assume a slightly lower absorption rate for some nutrients within multivitamins, as some will compete with others to be accepted. This *total* approach should be applied to all vitamins and minerals obtained from food, the sun, and supplements. Train yourself not to view supplemental vitamins and minerals in a vacuum. Consider all sources.

As of January 2021, you will find supplemental vitamin D amounts listed in micrograms (mcg) instead of international units (IU). Common values include vitamin D 25 mcg (1,000 IU), vitamin D 50 mcg (2,000 IU), and vitamin D 125 mcg (5,000 IU). One IU equals 0.025 mcg.

The following schedules are based on Life Extension Two-Per-Day multivitamins. Individuals may even consider breaking one tablet in half, to take two separate doses (breakfast and lunch) from one pill.

Table 20. Daily Supplement Schedule Ages 60+

	Breakfast	Lunch	Dinner	Optional^
Sun.	Magnesium 100–200 mg	Iodine 125–250 mcg	Magnesium 100–200 mg Copper 2 mg	Calcium 200–300 mg
Mon.	Multivitamin Magnesium 100–200 mg D3 50 mcg	K2 90–250 mcg Calcium 200–300 mg	Magnesium 100–200 mg Zinc 10–25 mg	
Tues.	Multivitamin Magnesium 100–200 mg	K2 90–250 mcg	Magnesium 100–200 mg Zinc 10–25 mg	
Wed.	Multivitamin Magnesium 100–200 mg D3 50 mcg	K2 90–250 mcg Calcium 200–300 mg	Magnesium 100–200 mg	Iodine 125–250 mcg
Thurs.	Multivitamin Magnesium 100–200 mg	K2 90–250 mcg	Magnesium 100–200 mg Zinc 10–25 mg	Calcium 200–300 mg
Fri.	Multivitamin Magnesium 100–200 mg D3 50 mcg	K2 90–250 mcg Calcium 200–300 mg	Magnesium 100–200 mg Zinc 10–25 mg	
Sat.	Magnesium 100–200 mg		Magnesium 100–200 mg	Multi-vitamin

NOTE: This schedule provides a comprehensive approach for individuals this age. However, the daily supplement schedule for ages 35–44 is my minimum recommendation for this age group.

^ Optional: You can add any or all supplements listed here to your weekly schedule.

Table 21. Daily Supplement Schedule Ages 45–59

	Breakfast	Lunch	Dinner	Optional^
Sun.	Magnesium 100–200 mg	Iodine 125–250 mcg Calcium 200–300 mg	Magnesium 100–200 mg	
Mon.	Multivitamin Magnesium 100–200 mg	K2 90–250 mcg Calcium 200–300 mg D3 25–50 mcg	Magnesium 100–200 mg Zinc 10–25 mg	
Tues.	Multivitamin Magnesium 100–200 mg	K2 90–250 mcg Calcium 200–300 mg	Magnesium 100–200 mg Zinc 10–25 mg	
Wed.	Multivitamin Magnesium 100–200 mg	K2 90–250 mcg D3 25–50 mcg	Magnesium 100–200 mg	Calcium 200–300 mg
Thurs.	Multivitamin Magnesium 100–200 mg	K2 90–250 mcg Calcium 200–300 mg	Magnesium 100–200 mg Zinc 10–25 mg	Iodine 125–250 mcg
Fri.	Multivitamin Magnesium 100–200 mg	K2 90–250 mcg Calcium 200–300 mg D3 25–50 mcg	Magnesium 100–200 mg Zinc 10–25 mg	
Sat.	Magnesium 100–200 mg		Magnesium 100–200 mg	Calcium 200–300 mg

NOTE: This schedule provides a comprehensive approach for individuals this age. However, the daily supplement schedule for ages 25–34 is my minimum recommendation for this age group.

^ Optional: You can add any or all supplements listed here to your weekly schedule.

Table 22. Daily Supplement Schedule Ages 35–44

	Breakfast	Lunch	Dinner	Optional^
Sun.	Iodine 125–250 mcg		Magnesium 100–200 mg	Calcium 200–300 mg
Mon.	Multivitamin Magnesium 100–200 mg	K2 90–250 mcg Calcium 200–300 mg	Magnesium 100–200 mg Zinc 10–25 mg	
Tues.	Multivitamin D3 25–50 mcg	K2 90–250 mcg	Magnesium 100–200 mg	
Wed.	Multivitamin Magnesium 100–200 mg	K2 90–250 mcg Calcium 200–300 mg	Magnesium 100–200 mg Zinc 10–25 mg	
Thurs.	Multivitamin D3 25–50 mcg	K2 90–250 mcg	Magnesium 100–200 mg	Iodine 125–250 mcg
Fri.	Multivitamin Magnesium 100–200 mg	K2 90–250 mcg Calcium 200–300 mg	Magnesium 100–200 mg Zinc 10–25 mg	
Sat.	D3 25–50 mcg		Magnesium 100–200 mg	Multivitamin

NOTE: This schedule provides a comprehensive approach for individuals this age. However, the daily supplement schedule for ages 25–34 is my minimum recommendation for this age group.

^ Optional: You can add any or all supplements listed here to your weekly schedule.

Table 23. Daily Supplement Schedule Ages 25–34

	Breakfast	Lunch	Optional^
Sun.			
Mon.	Multivitamin Magnesium 100–200 mg D3 25–50 mcg	Calcium 200–300 mg K2 90–250 mcg	Iodine 125–250 mcg
Tues.	Multivitamin Magnesium 100–200 mg	Calcium 200–300 mg	Zinc 10–25 mg
Wed.	Multivitamin Magnesium 100–200 mg D3 25–50 mcg	Calcium 200–300 mg K2 90–250 mcg	
Thurs.	Multivitamin Magnesium 100–200 mg Iodine 100–400 mcg*	Calcium 200–300 mg	Zinc 10–25 mg
Fri.	Multivitamin Magnesium 100–200 mg D3 25–50 mcg	Calcium 200–300 mg K2 90–250 mcg	
Sat.	Magnesium 100–200 mg	Calcium 200–300 mg	Zinc 10–25 mg

^ *Optional: You can add any or all supplements listed here to your weekly schedule.*

Table 24. Daily Supplement Schedule Ages 18–24

	Breakfast or Lunch	Optional but Recommended^
Sun.		
Mon.	Multivitamin Magnesium 100–200 mg	D3 25–50 mcg
Tues.	Multivitamin Magnesium 100–200 mg	Iodine 125–250 mcg
Wed.	Multivitamin Magnesium 100–200 mg	D3 25–50 mcg
Thurs.	Multivitamin Magnesium 100–200 mg	
Fri.	Multivitamin Magnesium 100–200 mg	D3 25–50 mcg
Sat.		Multivitamin

^ *Optional: You can add any or all supplements listed here to your weekly schedule. As stated previously, starting January 2021, you will find supplemental vitamin D amounts listed in micrograms (mcg) instead of international units (IU). Common values include vitamin D 25 mcg (1,000 IU), vitamin D 50 mcg (2,000 IU), and vitamin D 125 mcg (5,000 IU). One IU equals 0.025 mcg.*

PRODUCT LIST

Below is a list of products and manufacturers discussed in the preceding chapters. Although these are brands, I have come to trust, you may find others more to your liking.

As mentioned previously, it is better to purchase products from an actual vitamin store or directly from the manufacturer's website. Otherwise, be vigilant when buying vitamins through third-party internet retailers. The problem is not with the retailer; rather, there are issues with some of the sellers who use them.

It is worth repeating that there have been instances of sellers shipping counterfeit products. There have also been instances of sellers shipping expired or nearly expired products. This does not happen often, but it does warrant concern.

Make sure to read reviews for the seller. Examine the product and the expiration date. Some sellers have even stooped to covering expiration dates with barcode labels. Do not become frightened, but do be careful.

MAGNESIUM

Form:

- Magnesium glycinate (calming effect that may aid sleep)
- Magnesium citrate
- Magnesium aspartate
- Magnesium taurate

Product:

- Swanson—Chelated magnesium bisglycinate (133 mg)
- Whole Foods 365—Magnesium glycinate (~133 mg)
- Now Foods—Magnesium citrate (200 mg)
- Good State—Ionic (liquid) magnesium (100 mg)
- Doctor's Best—Chelated magnesium glycinate (100 mg)

VITAMIN K2

Form:

- Menaquinone—7 (MK-7)
- Product:
- Jarrow Formulas—MK-7 (90 mcg)
- Sports Research—MK-7 (100 mcg)

- Now Foods—MK-7 (100 mcg)

ZINC

Form:

- Zinc orotate (absorbs exceptionally well)
- Zinc monomethionine (absorbs extremely well)
- Zinc picolinate (absorbs extremely well; may upset an empty stomach)
- Zinc citrate (absorbs well; may upset an empty stomach)
- Zinc gluconate (absorbs well; may upset an empty stomach)

Product:

- Jarrow Formulas—Zinc Balance: Zinc (15 mg) copper (1 mg)
- Swanson—Zinc orotate (10 mg)
- Whole Foods 365—Zinc (15 mg) copper (1 mg)
- Solgar—Zinc picolinate (22 mg)
- Pure Encapsulations—Zinc 30: zinc picolinate (30 mg) (high dose, take less frequently)
- Kal—Zinc orotate (30 mg) (high dose, take less frequently)
- Liquid ionic zinc (various brands) (15 mg)

VITAMIN D

Form:

- D3

Product:

- Life Extension—D3 25 mcg (1,000 IU)
- Jarrow Formulas—D3 62.5 mcg (2,500 IU)
- Sports Research—D3 50 mcg (2,000 IU)

CALCIUM

Form:

- Calcium citrate (absorbs well with or without food)
- Calcium carbonate (take with food)

Product:

- Citracal Petites—Calcium citrate (200 mg) D3 (250 IU)
- Pure Encapsulations—Calcium citrate (150 mg)
- Bluebonnet—Calcium citrate (250 mg) D3 (200 IU) mag. aspartate (100 mg)
- NATURELO—Plant-based calcium (150 mg) D3 (6.25 mcg) mag. glycinate (50 mg)

IODINE

Form:

- Nascent (atomic) iodine (absorbs exceptionally well)
- Molecular iodine (absorbs well on an empty stomach)
- Potassium iodide (absorbs moderately well)

Product:

- LL—Magnetic clay nascent iodine, 1 oz (400 mcg per drop)
- Go Nutrients—Iodine edge nascent iodine (~300 mcg per drop)
- NOW—Kelp caps (150 mcg)

POTASSIUM

Form:

- Potassium chloride
- Potassium citrate

Product:

- NoSalt—Potassium chloride (640 mg per 1/4 tsp)
- Morton Salt Substitute—Potassium chloride (690 mg per 1/4 tsp)
- NOW—Potassium chloride powder (365 mg per 1/8 tsp)
- NOW—Potassium citrate powder (448 mg per 1/4 tsp)

MULTIVITAMIN

Product (estimated cost* at half-dose usage):

- Xtend-Life Natural Products—Total Balance ($26/month)
- Douglas Laboratories—Ultra Preventive X ($43/month)
- NATURELO—Whole Food Multivitamin ($45/month full dose)
- Life Extension—Life Extension Mix ($30/month)
- Life Extension—Two-Per-Day ($5/month)**
- Optimum Nutrition—Opti-Men/Opti-Women ($5/month)**

*estimated cost as of December 12, 2020
**additional cost required due to need for more standalone vitamins

CHAPTER TWENTY-FIVE

SLEEP

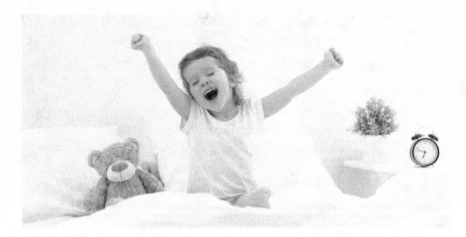

GETTING ADEQUATE SLEEP IS ONE of the most important steps you can take toward avoiding heart disease. Numerous studies demonstrate a dramatically increased risk for heart disease associated with chronic sleep deprivation.

Here is another little-known *secret*. When you sleep, your cardiovascular system enters a highly beneficial state called **nocturnal blood pressure (BP) dipping**. In this state, your blood pressure drops as much as 20 percent below your daytime resting state, relieving stress from your heart. Not achieving adequate sleep adversely impacts your ability to enter nocturnal BP dipping. A mere 5 percent reduction in nocturnal BP dipping resulted in roughly a 20-percent increase in death from cardiovascular events.[170,171,172]

Additionally, one study comprised of nearly 475,000 men and women revealed that individuals who regularly obtained less than six hours of sleep per night saw a 48 percent increase in developing coronary heart disease or suffering a fatal coronary event.[173]

Conversely, too much sleep also increases the risk of developing heart disease. Individuals who frequently sleep more than nine hours significantly increase the likelihood of developing calcium buildup in their arteries.

To maintain a healthy heart, individuals should obtain at least seven hours of sleep per night. Moreover, the quality of sleep is just as important as the duration. Habitually burning the midnight oil puts your heart at significant risk.[174]

"Insufficient sleep is associated with a number of chronic diseases and conditions—such as diabetes, cardiovascular disease, obesity, and depression—which threaten our nation's health."
—Centers for Disease Control and Prevention (CDC)

Taken daily but not together, 400 mg of calcium and 400 mg of magnesium is a natural cure for some forms of insomnia. However, calcium deposits may collect inside arteries when taken in excess. Therefore, obtain what you can from calcium-rich foods, such as milk and broccoli. I also do not recommend supplementing more than 250 mg in a single dose. As mentioned in previous chapters, it is imperative to maintain adequate levels of vitamin K2 to protect coronary arteries from calcium buildup. Please refer to Chapter 17 Calcium and Chapter 12 Magnesium for more details.

Chamomile tea also contains relaxing agents that can help

individuals to fall asleep. I caution against sleep aids such as melatonin unless used very sparingly. Individuals over sixty years of age may need supplemental melatonin because their bodies tend to produce less than nominal amounts. However, calcium naturally increases your body's melatonin production.[175]

BEDDING AND BREATHING

The better you breathe, the deeper you sleep. You also suffer from fewer sleep interruptions. Air quality can play a role in sleep quality, especially for those who suffer from certain allergies. Improving indoor air quality provides a host of benefits, including, for some, better sleep. As an asthma sufferer, I am personally aware of the impact indoor air quality has on my life. A few simple steps can make a world of difference.

Everyone should consider encasing their mattress inside a dust mite enclosure. Dust mites dine heavily on minute flakes of skin we shed. Places that may be overflowing with these flakes are mattresses and bedding. With current mattress technology and tightly woven fabric, dust mites may not be as invasive in some homes as they once were, but any reduction in their numbers can be beneficial. Seek high-end, breathable mattress covers. Pillows can be encased as well or periodically heated in a dryer.

Another superb return on investment to improve air quality are products like Filtrete HVAC filters. Filtrete filters are rated according to the size of the particles they can filter. The rating is based on a minimum efficiency reporting value (MERV). The higher the rating number, the greater the filtration. They even make *smart* filters that communicate via a phone app to alert you when to change them.

If your home is carpeted, a wise investment is a high-efficiency particulate air (HEPA) vacuum cleaner. HEPA rated filtration systems remove 99.97 percent of airborne particles that are 0.3 microns or larger across. Fortunately, the smallest bacteria are approximately 0.4 microns in size.

Household humidity should range from 30 percent up to 50 percent. When it drops toward 20 percent, your nasal passages and skin become drier and less pliable. You may find yourself scratching more frequently. In contrast, as humidity nears 60 percent, it becomes a breeding ground for mold, dust mites, and bacteria. It may be prudent to invest in a humidifier for use during the winter months and a dehumidifier for use during the summer if you reside in a humid region.

One costly investment that may be out of range for some households is replacing carpeting with tile or hardwood flooring. I replaced the carpet throughout the main floor, leaving the second floor carpeted. The difference in air quality is amazing! If installing flooring throughout your home is too expensive, consider only replacing the carpeting inside your bedroom to reduce allergens where you sleep.

EXERCISE

Exercise improves sleep and can be very beneficial for your heart. Resistance training forces your bones and muscles to adapt and grow denser. Try to make time to exercise four or five days a week, even if it means taking a brisk walk. Taking a full week off every fifth or sixth week should not hurt your progress. Ensure to follow the supplement schedule for your age group for better results. Using proper posture and technique will yield much better results than tossing extremely heavy weights into the air. Individuals suffering from bone conditions such as osteoporosis should avoid dynamic abdominal exercises like sit-ups and excessive twisting movements.

LIGHT

Blue light exposure up to two hours before or during sleep lowers melatonin production and shifts the circadian rhythm, which can adversely impact your rest. Digital clocks should contain red light displays and set to the lowest brightness setting. Night-lights should emit red light versus white or blue. Also, consider wearing glasses designed to block blue light when viewing computer screens, smartphones, or television within two hours before going to sleep.

Multi-color, smart LED bulbs may be a welcomed addition to the home. These amazing bulbs emit a broad array of colors, which are controlled by a smart-phone app. Individuals can also choose to enable voice commands via Siri, Alexa, or Google. They can even be programmed to change colors and intensity at various times each day. Moreover, they are extremely energy efficient.

CHAPTER TWENTY-SIX

ANXIETY AND STRESS

ANXIETY DISORDERS HAVE LONG BEEN associated with the early-onset and progression of cardiovascular health issues. Multiple studies associate stress, anxiety, and depression with heart failure, heart attacks, and death. High levels of anxiety were linked to a 44 percent increased risk of stroke, and 30 percent increased risk of heart attack.[176]

Following the global outbreak of an infectious contagion, COVID-19, hundreds of millions of individuals in the US and abroad were forced into extreme living conditions in hopes of mitigating the spread of the novel coronavirus. Consequently, millions of individuals lost their jobs and businesses, and children were forced out of their schools. Toilet paper, of all things, became a rare commodity, indicative of the stress and anxiety generated by the crisis.

Detailed studies are needed to assess the potentially far-reaching effects on stress, anxiety, and depression resulting from the pandemic and associated mitigation strategies. Additionally, COVID-19 post-traumatic stress disorder (PTSD) should be a real concern. Society may be dealing with the mental-health aftermath for years, if not decades to come. Mental health and economic challenges can negatively influence rates of obesity, substance abuse, and depression. These conditions adversely affect heart health.

Even though more research is needed to establish the full extent of the impact of anxiety and stress on the heart's health, scientists are generally in agreement that some of the answers lie in the endocrine system. The endocrine system regulates all hormonal functions in the body. In the face of a stressful situation, the human body is wired to either *defend itself* or *seek safety*—also known as the fight-or-flight response. This survival mechanism is facilitated by adrenal glands' release of the hormones adrenaline and cortisol.

THE ADRENALINE AND CORTISOL EFFECT

When adrenaline is released into the bloodstream, the heart rate and blood pressure subsequently increase to nourish the muscles for energy and the ability to contract in preparation to either fight or escape.

Cortisol, on the other hand, enhances the body and mind's learning and cognitive function. This helps the person to quickly learn, adapt, and recall how to respond to a stressful event from past experiences. The survival benefits of these reactions are obvious.

However, when stress and anxiety are prolonged or too recurrent, the body is constantly in a fight-or-flight survival mode, generating an overproduction of adrenaline and cortisol, potentially leading to severe hormonal imbalance.

In a study by researchers at a university hospital in Regensburg, Germany, hormonal imbalance of this nature was linked to increased inflammation in arteries.[177] The Department of Pharmacology at the University of São Paulo noted similar effects of hormonal imbalance and inflammation.[178] In addition to arterial inflammation, diminished hormonal regulation has been found to cause plaque buildup in arteries.[179] These conditions lay the groundwork for heart disease risk factors such as diabetes, hardening of the arteries, and high blood pressure.

RAPID HEART RATE (TACHYCARDIA) AND ABNORMAL HEART RHYTHMS (ARRHYTHMIA)

When facing a sudden stressful situation, there is an almost immediate sudden increase in heart rate. If the stressful event is resolved quickly, the heart rate drops without any severe consequences. However, when prolonged, anxiety and stress can lead to abnormal heart rhythms and possibly heart attacks.

HOPELESSNESS

Some researchers have identified a correlation between a prolonged sense of hopelessness and an increased risk of cardiovascular disease.[180,181] Due to the complexities surrounding this sensitive subject, individuals suffering from anxiety or a profound feeling of hopelessness will find a list of resources at the end of this chapter.

COPING STRATEGIES

The Anxiety and Depression Association of America (ADAA) provides a wealth of information on this subject. Tips they offer when you are feeling anxious or stressed include:[182]

> **"Take a time-out.** Practice yoga, listen to music, meditate, get a massage, or learn relaxation techniques. Stepping back from the problem helps clear your head.
>
> **Eat well-balanced meals.** Do not miss out on any meals. Do keep healthful, energy-boosting snacks on hand.
>
> **Limit alcohol and caffeine**, which can aggravate anxiety and trigger panic attacks.

> **Accept that you cannot control everything**. Put your stress in perspective: Is it as bad as you think?"

A comprehensive list of strategies is provided on the ADAA website at https://adaa.org/tips (URL is subject to change).

TOXIC RELATIONSHIPS

Toxic relationships play a significant role in heart disease. One study found a 34 percent risk increase of heart attack or chest pain in individuals living with a toxic relationship.[183] Many people know they are in a relationship with a toxic person yet find it difficult to dissolve the relationship for various reasons.

Toxic individuals care more about their own desires than the harm they inflict on others' lives. They are devious, self-serving, and unapologetic—except when being manipulative. Toxic people put you on the defensive and look toward others to solve their problems. Moreover, they selfishly take far more from a person than they are willing to give. They view kindness as a trait to take advantage of versus a quality to cherish. Your health and well-being are not a priority unless it serves their agenda. Your selflessness will not change their behavior; they go through life seeking individuals to benefit from or abuse.

Toxic individuals come in many forms. The stress or anxiety they ultimately bring into your life puts you at greater risk of developing heart disease and many other ailments, including depression. They will drain you financially or emotionally and interfere with your personal and professional goals. There are few conditions worse for your heart health and mental well-being than a toxic person. Lower your cardiovascular disease risk by identifying and removing toxic individuals from your personal life. These individuals are chameleons. Once they slither their way into your life, they may say anything to keep you or to damage your reputation once you are rid of them.

With the exception of toxic people, when you identify individuals in your life that may unknowingly raise your stress and anxiety levels, ask yourself what is it about the person that causes you to feel stressed or anxious? Determine if engaging in an open and honest conversation with the person may resolve or mitigate the issue(s). If they are unwilling or unable to modify their behavior, consider the following options:

- Examine yourself to ensure you are not overreacting. If you are, explore possible remedies, including professional counseling.
- Limit your exposure to these and similar individuals. Keep interactions brief and to the point.
- If their behavior crosses certain boundaries, such as harassment, seek legal recourse.
- Move on with your life. Weigh pros and cons for making significant changes, such as changing jobs or relocating. Make the best decision for you and your future. At times, it is okay to make yourself the priority.

Several years ago, I applied for and was promoted to a position at a somewhat prestigious training academy. This was my third application in five years, which made my acceptance very exuberating. Upon arrival, for reasons I cannot fathom, one manager, whom I did not work under, expressed disdain toward me. Whenever we found each other alone, he made demeaning remarks. One day, unsolicited, his secretary informed me this individual did not like me. She did not know what was wrong with him and suggested jealousy played a role in his attitude toward me.

One week later, my antagonist offered another negative comment as we crossed paths, which was the final straw. I considered expressing to him my willingness to beat him into an intensive care unit, which I was very capable of doing. Instead, I decided to speak with a union representative to understand the options in my new work environment. After careful consideration, I approached my branch manager and explained the situation. I informed him that if that individual made one more derogatory remark toward me, I would file a harassment complaint against him. As with many antagonists, the individual's behavior toward me was entirely unprovoked.

After explaining the issue to my manager, the antagonist never said another derogatory thing to me. I went on to thrive in my new position and career. I looked forward to going to work each day and enjoyed the social and professional interaction. Working at the academy was one of many challenging and rewarding positions I have had the privilege to serve.

This example demonstrates one of several methods one may adopt to reduce or eliminate stress. Life isn't solely based on what happens to us. Our reaction to situations and events can have a major positive or negative impact. Situations such as the one I encountered helped me understand the meaning of, *Don't let anyone steal your joy.* An antagonist attempted to steal my joy by creating a hostile work environment. I stopped him. So can you.

RELIGION

> "Most studies have shown that religious involvement and spirituality are associated with better health outcomes, including greater longevity, coping skills, and health-related quality of life (even during terminal illness) and less anxiety, depression, and suicide."
>
> **—Mayo Clinic Proceedings**

As indicated by the Mayo Clinic, several studies demonstrate a correlation between active religious involvement and better mental and physical health.[184] Moreover, studies further display a correlation between individuals who regularly attend religious services and a significantly decreased risk of cardiovascular disease. For example, a meta-analysis conducted in 2019 compared coronary heart disease (CHD) risk associated with attending religious services (R/S) once per month, to risk associated with attending religious services five times per month.[185]

> "The relative risks of CHD were 0.77 (CI 95% 0.65–0.91) for one-time attendance and 0.27 (CI 95% 0.11–0.65) for five-time attendance per month. R/S was associated with a significantly decreased risk of CHD."

Whether one believes in a divine creator or not, the preponderance of evidence indicating that regular attendance of religious services lowers your risk of heart disease cannot be ignored. Moreover, in the US, peer-reviewed studies conclude those who believe in a divine creator live an average of more than four years longer than nonbelievers.

Some individuals may seek secular reasons for the findings. Others may attribute them to the keeping of a divine promise.[186] In the end, it is up to everyone to decide what to believe for themselves.

MENTAL HEALTH RESOURCES

If you or someone you know is going through a stressful time or experiencing anxiety or depression, you are not alone. If you do not feel comfortable confiding with someone you know, multiple resources are at your disposal. Rather than toughing it out or suffering in silence, I implore you to reach out to one or several of the resources listed below. Please note that website addresses and phone numbers are subject to change.

American Psychiatric Association Foundation—Find a Psychiatrist: http://finder.psychiatry.org/

American Academy of Child and Adolescent Psychiatry—Child and Adolescent Psychiatrist Finder https://www.aacap.org

American Psychological Association—Find a Psychologist https://locator.apa.org

Veterans Crisis Line—1-800-273-TALK (8255)

Veterans Crisis Chat—text: 8388255

Department of Health & Human Services—SAMHSA's National Helpline—1-800-662-HELP (4357)

CHAPTER TWENTY-SEVEN

MEDICATIONS, SURGERY, AND TESTING

DEPENDING ON THE NATURE AND severity of a person's cardiovascular condition, your health-care provider may recommend prescription drugs. Examples listed here are generic names.

BLOOD-THINNING MEDICATION (ANTICOAGULANTS)

Blood thinners reduce the blood's clotting ability, also known as **coagulation**. In addition to preventing the formation of clots, they stop existing clots from growing larger. Doctors may prescribe a blood thinner to prevent stroke. These are common examples of anticoagulants:[187]

- Rivaroxaban
- Edoxaban
- Warfarin
- Apixaban

ANTIPLATELET AGENTS

These drugs reduce the tendency of blood platelets to stick together, consequently preventing the formation of clots. They can be prescribed as a preventive measure or to people who suffered heart attacks. Common antiplatelet drugs include:

- Aspirin
- Prasugrel
- Clopidogrel

ANGIOTENSIN-CONVERTING \ENZYME (ACE) INHIBITORS

ACE inhibitors are designed to improve blood circulation by decreasing resistance and expanding blood vessels. As a result, the heart does not need to exert as much force to pump blood throughout the body. Commonly prescribed ACE Inhibitors include:

- Fosinopril
- Moexipril
- Benazepril
- Ramipril

ANGIOTENSIN II RECEPTOR BLOCKERS (ARBS)

In simple terms, angiotensin II is a chemical present in the blood that increases blood pressure. ARBs are designed to neutralize the effects of angiotensin II, thereby keeping blood pressure levels optimal. Some common ARBs include:

- Candesartan
- Losartan
- Azilsartan

BETA-BLOCKERS

This medication lowers the heart rate and reduces the force of contraction. Consequently, the heart becomes subjected to less strain. They are prescribed to people with high blood pressure and abnormal heart rhythms. They include:

- Atenolol
- Metoprolol
- Propranolol

CALCIUM CHANNEL BLOCKERS

This medication works in two primary ways:

- Relax blood vessels
- Prevent calcium from entering blood vessels and the heart

Calcium channel blockers are prescribed to people with high blood pressure and chest pain (angina). They include:

- Felodipine (Plendil)
- Amlodipine (Norvasc)
- Nisoldipine (Sular)

SURGICAL PROCEDURES

Individuals may need to undergo surgery depending on the type and extent of cardiovascular disease they have. Some are more invasive and require more time to heal than others.

CORONARY ARTERY BYPASS GRAFTING (CABG)

CABG is a procedure done when there is some blockage in a coronary artery interrupting blood circulation. The surgeon identifies a healthy artery or vein from another part of your body and directly connects it to bypass the blockage and restore normal circulation.[188]

HEART VALVE REPAIR OR REPLACEMENT

This procedure repairs or replaces a valve. Replacements can either be artificial or derived from animal tissue.

ANGIOPLASTY (PERCUTANEOUS CORONARY INTERVENTIONS)

This procedure is performed to reverse a blockage or reduced blood flow in an artery. Once the surgeon identifies the blockage, they insert a special tubing along a coronary artery. This tubing contains an inflatable balloon at the tip, which will expand the blocked area to resume normal blood flow.[189] This often coincides with a tiny mesh coil (stent) placement.

Additional procedures are available. For more details, consult with your physician.

TESTS FOR HEART ATTACK

The risk of developing a heart attack can be determined through the following tests.

ECG TEST (EKG TEST)

The electrocardiogram is used to estimate the extent of damage to your heart muscle over the years. It also monitors heart rhythm and heart rate.

BLOOD TESTS

Cardiac enzymes are found within the heart. Their presence in the bloodstream indicates some form of heart muscle damage. Doctors can also measure the level of the protein Troponin in the blood. These proteins are usually released when heart cells are damaged due to a lack of blood supply.

ECHOCARDIOGRAPHY

Imaging is used to determine the pumping rhythm and activity of your heart. It incorporates an echo-based technique to tell whether various heart structures have been damaged.

TESTS FOR CARDIAC ARREST

No test can determine with 100 percent assurance whether or not a person will suffer cardiac arrest. However, there are a few tests that can be accomplished to assess the primary risk factors for cardiac arrest. In other words, the likelihood of someone suffering a cardiac arrest event can be determined to a degree by a combination of family history, lifestyle, current health condition, and the following tests.

CARDIAC CATHETERIZATION

This test is conducted by an interventional cardiologist who uses a catheter (tube) inserted into a blood vessel to inspect the nature of your heart issues.

ECHOCARDIOGRAPHY

This imaging test allows the doctor to create computerized pictures of your heart and its attached blood vessels. From here, the doctor can inspect and assess the health and condition of your heart and abnormalities, if any.

NUCLEAR CARDIOLOGY IMAGING

This is a noninvasive procedure that uses minimal amounts of radioactive material to map out the heart and its various parts. The doctor can then assess the extent of heart damage and the likelihood of cardiac arrest.

As stated earlier, there are many forms of heart disease. The focus of this information is on the most prevalent forms of heart disease over which you have the power to influence.

TESTS FOR ENDOTHELIAL FUNCTION

Medical technology has dramatically advanced over the years providing options to measure endothelial function.[190]

CORONARY FLOW RESERVE TEST

This test involves injecting dilating chemicals into specific blood vessels, followed by close monitoring of blood pressure. A lack of proper decreased blood flow from induced dilation is enough to indicate a possible endothelial dysfunction. This is an invasive procedure. Less-invasive methods are available.

FLOW-MEDIATED DILATION (FMD)

This common method utilizes an ultrasound of the brachial artery to measure the amount of dilation (width of the interior passageway) inside, along with other parameters.

PHASE-CONTRAST MAGNETIC RESONANCE IMAGING

As a noninvasive approach, this test uses magnetic imaging to monitor blood flow velocities in the arteries. Monitoring flow provides an insight into the state of the endothelial walls.

POSITRON EMISSION TOMOGRAPHY (PET SCAN)

Next in our noninvasive testing methods is a PET scan, which produces identifiable imaging by detecting photons emitted in blood vessel tissue. Many reports have similarly found this to be a useful way of monitoring endothelial function.

CONCLUSION

NUTRIENTS AFFECT EVERY ASPECT OF your health, including heart health. The state of your health affects every part of your life. Every few years, a new wonder-diet goes viral, causing multitudes of *experts* to flood the internet with blogs and forums. They claim to have found the diet or the superfood we have all been searching for (until the next one comes along). They blame entire food groups for all that ails humanity. Unfortunately, they focus too heavily on quick fixes without considering long-term risks.

There are no miracle pills or miracle foods for long-term health. Apart from unique situations, optimal balance leads to optimal health. Regardless of the dietary path you choose, peak heart health and performance begins at the cellular level. Give your cells and organs the proper balance of nutrients they need to flourish; in turn, they will optimize your cardiovascular fitness throughout your life. We are all complex and unique organisms. Your cells and organs need the right combination of raw materials to construct and maintain that complex and unique structure that is *you*.

The focus of this information has not been on extreme measures or dramatic lifestyle changes. Rather, it is on basic, key steps to prevent or mitigate heart disease, high blood pressure, and other health-related issues. Genetics is something we have little control over. At best, we can avoid things that mutate our DNA or aggravate genetic conditions. However, runners, weightlifters, cyclists, and couch potatoes can improve their cardiovascular health by reversing nutrient deficiencies, removing nutrient excess, and maintaining healthy organs. Nutrient balance obtained via vitamin therapy can also reduce dependency on costly prescription drugs. The endothelium, liver, and nocturnal BP dipping are rarely included in discussions involving heart health. As you discovered, they are primary factors in maintaining a healthy heart and extending one's life. The information contained here has worked wonders for myself, my loved ones, and my colleagues. Now, it can work for you.

The material you have just read addresses several of the more commonly overlooked deficiencies in industrialized nations. Resolving them affords you major health gains for the smallest investments. You do not have to start running marathons. Rather, you only need to add a few vitamins, foods, or drinks to your diet. That said, running marathons can be an interesting challenge and a lot of fun!

This is your opportunity to improve your health and performance at the cardiovascular cellular level. This is your opportunity to offer your cells the environment they need to build and maintain an even stronger and healthier you. Give yourself the gift of optimal heart health. Be patient. Be consistent. Be cheerful. Most importantly, be well!

SHARE THE HEALTH

Other books by Bryant Lusk.

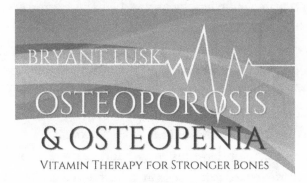
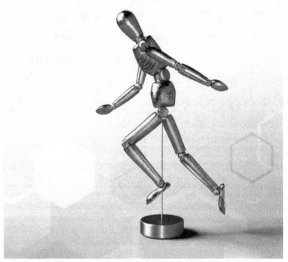

USEFUL TERMS

Adequate Intake (AI) levels are established when there is not enough documented evidence to develop an RDA. AI is set at a level assumed to ensure nutritional adequacy. AI is based on observed intakes of the nutrient by a group of healthy persons.

Bioavailability is a term used to identify the ease or difficulty by which a nutrient is absorbed into your system. High bioavailability means your body will readily absorb more of the nutrient.

Buffering a substance reduces its potential to irritate your digestive system through symptoms such as nausea or diarrhea. Buffering will make a substance either less alkaline or less acidic.

Chelation is a method of binding a substance to a protein to increase its bioavailability. Binding a substance to a protein greatly increases its absorption rate.

Dietary Reference Intakes (DRIs) are based on multiple reference values: Adequate Intake (AI), Recommended Dietary Allowance (RDA), Tolerable Upper Intake Level (UL).

Estimated Average Requirement (EAR) is the amount of a nutrient that is estimated to meet the requirement of half of all healthy individuals in the population.

Gastrointestinal (GI) Transit Time is the amount of time required for food to pass through to your stool, which is 1.5–3 days on average. High-protein meals travel at a slower pace, allowing the protein to be absorbed more fully. The foods you eat are not expelled in the same order that you eat them. Some food elements are pushed past others.

Minerals serve a multitude of functions, are used to regulate heart rhythm and muscle contractions, build strong bones and teeth, regulate fluid inside and outside cells, create energy, and transfer electrical signals through your nervous system. Minerals that our bodies utilize are listed below:

Calcium, chloride, chromium, copper, fluoride, iodine, iron, magnesium, manganese, molybdenum, phosphorus, potassium, selenium, sodium, sulfur, zinc.

Recommended Dietary Allowance (RDA) is the daily level of intake sufficient to meet the nutrient requirements of nearly all (97–98 percent) healthy individuals. The RDA is often set at the lower end of the full range of what individuals can tolerate before a nutrient becomes unsafe.

Tolerable Upper Intake Level (UL) is the maximum daily intake unlikely to cause harm.

Vitamins (Fat Soluble) are ingested from animal fats, butter, vegetable oils, dairy, fish, and liver. The human body is very effective at storing these vitamins in your liver and fatty tissues for future use. If you regularly consume more than you need (mega-dose), some fat-soluble vitamins can damage your organs, nervous system, and brain. Fat-soluble vitamins remain available even after foods containing them are cooked. They absorb best with meals containing healthy fats (e.g., flaxseed, olive oil, eggs, avocados, lake herring, lake trout, mackerel, wild salmon, sardines, and tuna).

Fat-soluble vitamins are vitamins A, D, E, and K.

Vitamins (Water Soluble) are mainly sourced from fruits, vegetables, and grains and are not as resilient to heat as fat-soluble vitamins. Water-soluble vitamins are not stored for very long and need to be replenished more frequently. Excess is primarily excreted via your urine.

Water-soluble vitamins are vitamins C, biotin, B1 (thiamine), B2 (riboflavin), B6 (pyridoxine), niacin (nicotinic acid), B12, folic acid, and pantothenic acid.

ABOUT BRYANT LUSK

BRYANT LUSK IS A MILITARY veteran who grew up on the south side of Chicago. Despite the challenges of gang violence and poverty, he became a successful Safety Inspector and Quality Control Specialist with the United States Government.

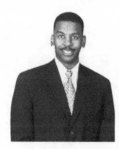 Bryant spent four years in the United States Air Force, learning the true meaning of empowerment and pride. His desire to serve and protect others led him to write the initial installment of his *Share the Health* book series. With a determination to treat debilitating conditions, Bryant's books have helped many.

With this latest offering, Bryant shifts the focus to naturally treating cardiovascular disease and hypertension, a set of conditions that inflicts pain and fatalities on millions of women and men worldwide. By identifying the best formulations of vitamins and minerals required to treat or prevent various causes of heart disease, his approach to vitamin therapy is both affordable and effective.

Bryant enjoys learning through cultural encounters and watching classic films. He particularly enjoys spending quality time with friends and loved ones, and of course, carrying out research and writing on the things that go toward helping millions of people to improve their health and quality of life.

> *"I measure success by the number of people that I affect in a positive and meaningful way."*
>
> **—Bryant Lusk**

ENDNOTES

[1] Benedict M, Zhang X. (2017 Jun. 8) Non-alcoholic fatty liver disease: An expanded review. World J Hepatol. doi: 10.4254/wjh.v9.i16.715

[2] Hunt CM, Turner MJ, Gifford EJ, et al. (2019) Identifying and treating nonalcoholic fatty liver disease. Fed Pract.

[3] Centers for Disease Control and Prevention: Heart Disease Statistics and Maps (Last Reviewed 2019-Dec. 02) https://www.cdc.gov/heartdisease/facts.htm.

[4] Rakesh K. Pai, MD - Cardiology, Electrophysiology & Anne C. Poinier, MD - Internal Medicine & Martin J. Gabica, MD - Family Medicine & Adam Husney, MD - Family Medicine & Stephen Fort, MD, MRCP, FRCPC - Interventional Cardiology, MyHealth.Alberta.Ca (2018): "How the Heart Works"

[5] Mozaffarian D, Benjamin EJ, Go AS, et al. Heart Disease and Stroke Statistics—2015 update: a report from the American Heart Association. Circulation 2015; 131:e29-322

[6] Harvard Health Publishing, Harvard Medical School (Last Updated 2015-07) Race and ethnicity: Clues to your heart disease risk

[7] Hagström H, Nasr P, Ekstedt M, et al. (2019 Jan.) Cardiovascular risk factors in non-alcoholic fatty liver disease. Liver Int. doi: 10.1111/liv.13973

[8] Claudio Tana,1 Stefano Ballestri,2 Fabrizio Ricci, et al. (2019 Sep.) Cardiovascular Risk in Non-Alcoholic Fatty Liver Disease: Mechanisms and Therapeutic Implications. Int J Environ Res Public Health. doi: 10.3390/ijerph16173104

[9] American Heart Association, (Last Reviewed 2019) Understand Your Risks to Prevent a Heart Attack

[10] American Heart Association (Last Reviewed 2018-03) Heart Disease and Stroke Statistics—2018 Update: A Report from the American Heart Association. Circulation 2018; 137:e67–e492

[11] Félétou M, San R (2011) The Endothelium: Part 1: Multiple Functions of the Endothelial Cells—Focus on Endothelium-Derived Vasoactive Mediators. Morgan & Claypool Life Sciences. NBK57148

[12] Jay W, Amir L (2014 Oct.) Endothelial dysfunction and cardiovascular disease. Global Cardiology Science and Practice. doi: 10.5339/gcsp.2014.43.

[13] Jean D, Peter G (2004 June) Role of Endothelial Dysfunction in Atherosclerosis. Circulation. 109:III-27–III-32. doi: 10.1161/01. CIR.0000131515.03336.f8.

[14] Dimitris Tousoulis, Anna-Maria Kampoli, Costas Tentolouris, et. al. (2012 Jan). *The role of nitric oxide on endothelial function.* Current Vascular Pharmacology. doi: 10.2174/157016112798829760

[15] G. Walford J. Loscalzo (2003 Aug) *Nitric oxide in vascular biology.* Journal of Thrombosis and Haemostasis. doi: 10.1046/j.1538-7836.2003.00345.x

[16] R O Cannon 3rd (1998 Aug). Role of nitric oxide in cardiovascular disease: focus on the endothelium. Clin Chem.

[17] G J Dusting (1996) *Nitric oxide in coronary artery disease: roles in atherosclerosis, myocardial reperfusion and heart failure.* Karmazyn M. (eds) Myocardial Ischemia: Mechanisms, Reperfusion, Protection. EXS, vol 76. Birkhäuser Basel. doi: 10.1007/978-3-0348-8988-9_3

[18] Uffe Ravnskov 1, Michel de Lorgeril 2, David M Diamond, et al. (2018 Oct) LDL-C does not cause cardiovascular disease: a comprehensive review of the current literature. Expert Rev Clin Pharmacol. doi: 10.1080/17512433.2018.1519391

[19]   World Health Organization (WHO). (2019 Sep. 13). Hypertension. https://www.who.int/news-room/fact-sheets/detail/hypertension

[20]   Centers for Disease Control and Prevention (CDC). Hypertension Cascade: Hypertension Prevalence, Treatment and Control Estimates Among US Adults Aged 18 Years and Older Applying the Criteria From the American College of Cardiology and American Heart Association's 2017 Hypertension Guideline—NHANES 2013–2016

[21]   Centers for Disease Control and Prevention. Underlying Cause of Death, 1999–2018. CDC WONDER Online Database. Atlanta, GA: Centers for Disease Control and Prevention; 2018. http://wonder.cdc.gov/ucd-icd10.html. Accessed October 11, 2020.

[22]   Islam Bolad, Patrice Delafontaine. (2005 Jul). *Endothelial dysfunction: its role in hypertensive coronary disease.* Current Opinion in Cardiology. doi: 10.1097/01.hco.0000167719.37700.1d

[23]   J A Panza, A A Quyyumi, J E Brush Jr, et. al. (1990 Jul). *Abnormal Endothelium-Dependent Vascular Relaxation in Patients with Essential Hypertension.* New England Journal of Medicine. doi: 10.1056/NEJM199007053230105

[24]   Anthony M. Heagerty, et.al., (2010). *Small artery structure and function in hypertension.* Journal of Cellular and Molecular Medicine. doi: 10.1111/j.1582-4934.2010.01080.x

[25]   Yoshiteru Tada, MD, PhD, et.al., (2014) *Roles of hypertension in the rupture of intracranial aneurysms.* Department of Anesthesia and Perioperative Care, University of California, San Francisco. doi: 10.1161/STROKEAHA.113.003072

[26]   Rita Facchetti, et.al., (2019) High Normal Blood Pressure and Left Ventricular Hypertrophy Echocardiographic Findings From the PAMELA Population. Department of Medicine and Surgery, University of Milano-Bicocca, Italy. doi: 1161/HYPERTENSIONAHA.118.12114

[27]   R. Swaminathan (1986) Magnesium metabolism and its disorders. Clin Biochem Rev. 2003;24(2):47–66.

[28]   Saris NE, Mervaala E, Karppanen H, Khawaja JA, Lewenstam A. Magnesium. An update on physiological, clinical and analytical aspects. Clin Chim Acta. 2000;294:1–26.

[29]   Fox C, Ramsoomair D, Carter C. Magnesium: its proven and potential clinical significance. South Med J. 2001;94:1195–1201.

[30]   Swaminathan R. Magnesium metabolism and its disorders. Clin Biochem Rev. 2003;24(2):47–66.

[31]   Shechter M, Hod H, Marks N, Behar S, Kaplinsky E, Rabinowitz B. Beneficial effect of Magnesium sulfate in acute myocardial infarction. Am J Cardiol. 1990;66:271–274. doi: 10.1016/0002-9149(90)90834-.

[32]   Gu Wj, Wu Zj, Wang Pf, et al,. (2012 Apr). Intravenous magnesium prevents atrial fibrillation after coronary artery bypass grafting: a meta-analysis of 7 double-blind, placebo-controlled, randomized clinical trials. Trials. 2012;13:41. doi: 10.1186/1745-6215-13-41.

[33]   ANGUS M, ANGUS Z. Cardiovascular actions of magnesium. Crit Care Clin. 2001;53:299–307.

[34]   Haigney MC, Silver B, Tanglao E, et al. (1995 Oct 15) Noninvasive Measurement of Tissue Magnesium and Correlation with Cardiac Levels. Circulation. 92(8):2190-7.

[35]   Burton B. Silver, Ph.D. copyright 1980–2014. Non-invasive Intracellular Mineral-Electrolyte Analysis; Published Research and References, http://www.exatest.com/Research.htm.

[36]   Caroline Bell Stowe, (2011) *The effects of pomegranate juice consumption on blood pressure and cardiovascular health.* Complement Ther Clin Pract. doi: 10.1016/j.ctcp.2010.09.004

[37]   Claudio Ferri, et.al., Department of Life, Health & Environmental Sciences, University of L'Aquila, Italy (2017). *Effects of pomegranate juice on blood pressure: A systematic review and meta-analysis of randomized controlled trials.* Pharmacol Res. DOI: 10.1016/j.phrs.2016.11.018

[38]   Gemma Vilahur, et.al., Centro de Investigación Cardiovascular, CSIC-ICCC, Hospital de la Santa Creu i Sant Pau, IIB-Sant Pau, Barcelona, Spain, (2015):. *Polyphenol-enriched diet prevents coronary endothelial dysfunction by activating the Akt/eNOS pathway.* Rev Esp Cardiol (Engl Ed). DOI: 10.1016/j.rec.2014.04.021

[39]   Ahmad Esmaillzadeh, et.al., Department of Human Nutrition, National Nutrition and Food Technology Research Institute, Tehran, Iran, (2006). *"Cholesterol-lowering effect of concentrated pomegranate juice consumption in type II diabetic patients with hyperlipidemia.* Int J Vitam Nutr Res. DOI: 10.1024/0300-9831.76.3.147

[40]   Michael Aviram, et.al., (2000). Pomegranate juice consumption reduces oxidative stress, atherogenic modifications to LDL, and platelet aggregation: studies in humans and in atherosclerotic apolipoprotein E–deficient mice. American Journal of Clinical Nutrition. doi: 10.1093/ajcn/71.5.1062

[41]   Atheroma. (n.d.). In Wikipedia. Retrieved November 10, 2020, from https://en.wikipedia.org/wiki/Atheroma

[42]   Emad Al-Dujaili, Nacer Smail. (2012) Pomegranate juice intake enhances salivary testosterone levels and improves mood and well being in healthy men and women. Endocrine Abstracts.

[43]   E M Al-Olayan, M F El-Khadragy, D M Metwally, et al., (2014 May) Protective effects of pomegranate (Punica granatum) juice on testes against carbon tetrachloride intoxication in rats. BMC Complement Altern Med. doi: 10.1186/1472-6882-14-164

[44]   Gaffari Türk, Mustafa Sönmez, Muhterem Aydin, et al. (2008 Apr) Effects of pomegranate juice consumption on sperm quality, spermatogenic cell density, antioxidant activity and testosterone level in male rats. Clinical Nutrition. doi: 10.1016/j.clnu.2007.12.006

[45]   E M Al-Olayan, M F El-Khadragy, D M Metwally, et al., (2014 May) Protective effects of pomegranate (Punica granatum) juice on testes against carbon tetrachloride intoxication in rats. BMC Complement Altern Med. doi: 10.1186/1472-6882-14-164

[46]   Gaffari Türk, Mustafa Sönmez, Muhterem Aydin, et al. (2008 Apr) Effects of pomegranate juice consumption on sperm quality, spermatogenic cell density, antioxidant activity and testosterone level in male rats. Clinical Nutrition. doi: 10.1016/j.clnu.2007.12.006

[47]   Pandey KB, Rizvi SI. Plant polyphenols as dietary antioxidants in human health and disease. Oxidative Med Cell Longev. (2009) doi: 10.4161/oxim.2.5.9498

[48]   Ramírez-Garza, S. L., Laveriano-Santos E. P., Marhuenda-Muñoz M. et al. (2018 December) Health Effects of Resveratrol: Results from Human Intervention Trials. Nutrients. doi: 10.3390/nu10121892

[49]   Imamura H., Yamaguchi T., Nagayama D. et al. (2017 August) Resveratrol Ameliorates Arterial Stiffness Assessed by Cardio-Ankle Vascular Index in Patients With Type 2 Diabetes Mellitus. International Heart Journal, doi: 10.1536/ihj.16-373

[50]   Zhang J. et al (2017 May) *Resveratrol may reduce arterial stiffness in patients with diabetes.* Helioealio. https://www.healio.com/news/cardiology/20170504/resveratrol-may-reduce-arterial-stiffness-in-patients-with-diabetes

[51]   Theodotou M., Fokianos K., Mouzouridou A. et al. (2016 December) *The effect of resveratrol on hypertension: A clinical trial.* Experimental and Therapeutic Medicine, 13, 295-301. doi: 10.3892/etm.2016.3958

52   Tomé-Carneiro J., Gonzálvez M., Larrosa M. et al. (2012 April) One-Year Consumption of a Grape Nutraceutical Containing Resveratrol Improves the Inflammatory and Fibrinolytic Status of Patients in Primary Prevention of Cardiovascular Disease. The American Journal of Cardiology. doi: 10.1016/j.amjcard.2012.03.030

53   Tomé-Carneiro J., Gonzálvez M., Larrosa M. et al. (2012 May). Consumption of a grape extract supplement containing resveratrol decreases oxidized LDL and ApoB in patients undergoing primary prevention of cardiovascular disease: A triple-blind, 6-month follow-up, placebo-controlled, randomized trial. Molecular Nutrition & Food Research. doi:10.1002/mnfr.201100673

54   Mukherjee S., Dudley J.I., Das D.K. Dose-Dependency of Resveratrol in Providing Health Benefits. Dose-Response. 2010;8:478–500. doi: 10.2203/dose-response.09-015.Mukherjee.

55   Mankowski R.T., You L., Buford T.W., et al. (2020) Higher dose of resveratrol elevated cardiovascular disease risk biomarker levels in overweight older adults - A pilot study. Exp. Gerontol. doi: 10.1016/j.exger.2019.110821

56   K Magyar 1, R Halmosi, A Palfi, G Feher, et al.(2012) Cardioprotection by resveratrol: A human clinical trial in patients with stable coronary artery disease, IOS Press, doi: 10.3233/CH-2011-1424

57   Priyanka Chatterjee, et.al., (2012): Evaluation of anti-inflammatory effects of green tea and black tea: A comparative in vitro study. Journal of Advanced Pharmaceutical Technology & Research. doi: 10.4103/2231-4040.97298

58   Bradley J. Newsome, et.al., (2014). *Green tea diet decreases PCB 126-induced oxidative stress in mice by up-regulating antioxidant enzymes.* Journal of Nutritional Biochemistry. doi: 10.1016/j.jnutbio.2013.10.003

[59]   M. A. Islam. USA (2012). Cardiovascular Effects of Green Tea Catechins: Progress and Promise., LECOM School of Pharmacy. doi: 10.2174/157489012801227292

[60]   Pooja Bhardwaj an Deepa Khanna, Cardiovascular (2013). *Green tea catechins: defensive role in cardiovascular disorders.* Chinese Journal of Natural Medicines. doi: 10.1016/S1875-5364(13)60051-5

[61]   Jane E Freedman, MD (2019 July). *The role of platelets in coronary heart disease.* https://www.uptodate.com/contents/1498

[62]   Francesca Bravi, Carlo La Vecchia,corresponding, Federica Turati. (2017 April). Green tea and liver cancer. Hepatobiliary Surgery and Nutrition. doi: 10.21037/hbsn.2017.03.07

[63]   Elizabeth X Zheng, Simona Rossi, Robert J Fontana. (2016 Aug.). Risk of Liver Injury Associated with Green Tea Extract in SLIMQUICK(®) Weight Loss Products: Results from the DILIN Prospective Study. doi: 10.1007/s40264-016-0428-7

[64]   Jiang Hua, Donna Webster, Joyce Caoc, et al. (2018 Jun.). *The safety of green tea and green tea extract consumption in adults – Results of a systematic review.* Regulatory Toxicology and Pharmacology. doi: 10.1016/j.yrtph.2018.03.019

[65]   Yan Jin, Jing Zhao, Eun Mi Kim, et al. (2019 May). Comprehensive Investigation of the Effects of Brewing Conditions in Sample Preparation of Green Tea Infusions. Molecules. doi: 10.3390/molecules24091735

[66]   Loomis, Dana & Guyton, Kathryn & Grosse, et al,. (2016 June 15). *Carcinogenicity of drinking coffee, mate, and very hot beverages.* The Lancet. Oncology. doi: 10.1016/S1470-2045(16)30239-X.

[67]   Gast G.C., de Roos N.M., Sluijs I., et al. (2009 Sep.) A high menaquinone intake reduces the incidence of coronary heart disease. Nutr. Metab. Cardiovasc. Dis. 2009;19:504–510. doi: 10.1016/j.numecd.2008.10.004.

[68] Beulens JW, Bots ML, Atsma F. Marie-Louise E.L. et al. (2008 Jul 07). High dietary menaquinone intake is associated with reduced coronary calcification. *Atherosclerosis*, 203, Issue 2, 489–493.

[69] Schurgers LJ, Cranenburg EC, Vermeer C. (2008 Sep 5). Matrix Gla-protein: the calcification inhibitor in need of vitamin K. *Thrombosis and Haemostasis*. Thieme. doi: 10.1160/TH08-02-0087.

[70] Johanna M Geleijnse 1, Cees Vermeer, Diederick E Grobbee, et al,. (2004 Nov). Dietary intake of menaquinone is associated with a reduced risk of coronary heart disease: the Rotterdam Study. J Nutr. doi: 10.1093/jn/134.11.3100

[71] G C M Gast , N M de Roos, I Sluijs, et al. (2009 Sep). *A high menaquinone intake reduces the incidence of coronary heart disease.* Nutrition, Metabolism and Cardiovascular Diseases. doi: 10.1016/j.numecd.2008.10.004

[72] Shearer MJ. (2000 Nov). Role of vitamin K and Gla proteins in the pathophysiology of osteoporosis and vascular calcification. Current Opinion in Clinical Nutrition and Metabolic Care. doi: 10.1097/00075197-200011000-00004

[73] Szulc P, Arlot M, Chapuy MC, et al,. (1994 Oct). *Serum undercarboxylated osteocalcin correlates with hip bone mineral density in elderly women.* Journal of Bone and Mineral Research. doi: 10.1002/jbmr.5650091012.

[74] Knapen MH, Drummen NE, Smit E, Vermeer C, Theuwissen E. (2013 Sep 24). *Three-year low-dose menaquinone-7 supplementation helps decrease bone loss in healthy postmenopausal women.* Osteoporosis International. doi: 10.1007/s00198-013-2325-6.

[75] Juanola-Falgarona M, Salas-Salvadó J, Martínez-González MÁ, et al. (2014 May). Dietary intake of vitamin K is inversely associated with mortality risk. The American Institute of Nutrition—Journal of Nutrition.

[76]   Hans-Jürgen Apell, Tanja Hitzler and Grischa Schreiber, American Chemical Society (Last Reviewed 2017) Modulation of the Na,K-ATPase by Magnesium Ions. doi: 10.1021/acs.biochem.6b01243

[77]   Wilhelm Jahnen-Dechent and Markus Ketteler, Clinical Kidney Journal, Volume 5, Issue Suppl_1, February 2012, Pages i3–i14 (Last Updated 2012-02) Magnesium basics; doi: 10.1093/ndtplus/sfr163

[78]   Jeroen H. F. de Baaij, Joost G. J. Hoenderop, and René J. M. Bindels, American Journal of Hypertension (Last Updated 2009-07) Oral Magnesium Supplementation Reduces Ambulatory Blood Pressure in Patients With Mild Hypertension. doi: 10.1038/ajh.2009.126

[79]   L Kass, J Weekes & L Carpenter, European Journal of Clinical Nutrition (Last Updated 2012) Effect of magnesium supplementation on blood pressure: a meta-analysis. doi: 10.1038/ejcn.2012.4

[80]   Jeanette A.M.Maier, Molecular Aspects of Medicine, Volume 24, Issues 1–3, Pages 137-146 (Last Updated 2003) Low magnesium and atherosclerosis: an evidence-based link. https://doi.org/10.1016/S0098-2997(02)00095-X

[81]   Ko HJ, Youn CH, Kim HM, et al. (2014 Jun) Dietary Magnesium Intake and Risk of Cancer: A Meta-Analysis of Epidemiologic Studies. Thyroid Research Journal. 9:1-9.

[82]   Rivlin RS. Magnesium deficiency and alcohol intake: mechanisms, clinical significance, and possible relation to cancer development (a review). J Am Coll Nutr 1994;13:416–23.

[83]   Dean C. (2012 Jun 3). Magnesium – The Weight Loss Cure. Natural News. http://www.naturalnews.com/036049_magnesium_weight_loss_cure.html.

[84]   James J DiNicolantonio, Jing Liu and James H O'Keefe1, The BMJ (Last Updated 2018-07) Magnesium for the prevention and treatment of cardiovascular disease; doi: 10.1136/openhrt-2018-000775

[85] Nazanin Roohani, Richard Hurrell, Roya Kelishadi et al., (2013): "Zinc and its importance for human health: An integrative review." Retrieved from https://www.ncbi.nlm.nih.gov/pmc/articles/PMC3724376/

[86] Woodier J, Rainbow RD, Stewart AJ et al., (2015). *Intracellular Zinc Modulates Cardiac Ryanodine Receptor-mediated Calcium Release.* Journal of Biological Chemistry. DOI: https://doi.org/10.1074/jbc.M115.661280

[87] Turan B, Tuncay E, (2017 Nov): *"Impact of Labile Zinc on Heart Function: From Physiology to Pathophysiology.* Int J Mol Sci. DOI: 10.3390/ijms18112395

[88] Yoshihisa A, Abe S, Kiko T et al., (2018 Jun). *Association of Serum Zinc Level With Prognosis in Patients With Heart Failure.* J Card Fail. DOI: 10.1016/j.cardfail.2018.02.011

[89] Angel Lopez-Candales, Paula M. Hernández Burgos, Dagmar F. Hernandez-Suarez et al., (2017). *Linking Chronic Inflammation with Cardiovascular Disease: From Normal Aging to the Metabolic Syndrome.* J Nat Sci. https://www.ncbi.nlm.nih.gov/pmc/articles/PMC5488800/

[90] Ananda S.Prasad, (2014). Zinc: An antioxidant and anti-inflammatory agent: Role of zinc in degenerative disorders of aging. Doi: 10.1016/j.jtemb.2014.07.019

[91] Islamoglu Y, Evliyaoglu O, Tekbas E et al., (2011). *The relationship between serum levels of Zn and Cu and severity of coronary atherosclerosis.* Springer Link. Doi: 10.1007/s12011-011-9123-9

[92] Klevay L (1975) Coronary heart disease: the zinc/copper hypothesis. Am J Clin Nutr 28:764–774

[93] Perry DK, Smyth MJ, Stennicke HR et al (1997) Zinc is a potent inhibitor of the apoptotic protease, caspase-3. A novel target for zinc in the inhibition of apoptosis. J Biol Chem 272:18530–18533

[94]   Soinio M, Marniemi J, Laakso M et al (2007) Serum zinc level and coronary heart disease events in patients with type 2 diabetes. Diabetes Care 30:523–528

[95]   Kim J. (2013 Dec). Dietary zinc intake is inversely associated with systolic blood pressure in young obese women. *Nutrition Research and Practice.* 7(6):519.

[96]   Yamaguchi M. (2010 May). Role of nutritional zinc in the prevention of osteoporosis. *Molecular and Cellular Biochemistry.* 338(1-2):241-54. doi: 10.1007/s11010-009-0358-0.

[97]   Haase H, Rink L. (2009 June 12). The immune system and the impact of zinc during aging. *Immunity & Ageing.* 6: 9. doi: 10.1186/1742-4933-6-9.

[98]   Singh RB, Niaz MA, Rastogi SS, Bajaj S, et al. (1998 Dec). Current zinc intake and risk of diabetes and coronary artery disease and factors associated with insulin resistance in rural and urban populations of *North India. Journal of the American College of Nutrition.* 17(6):564-70.

[99]   Swardfager W. Ph.D , Herrmann N. M.D., Mazereeuw G. Ph.D Candidate, et al (2013 Dec 15). Zinc in Depression: A Meta-Analysis. *Biological Psychiatry.* 74, (12): 872–878.

[100]   Payahoo L, Ostadrahimi A, Mobasseri M, et al. (2013). Effects of Zinc Supplementation on the Anthropometric Measurements, Lipid Profiles and Fasting Blood Glucose in the Healthy Obese Adults. *Advanced Pharmaceutical Bulletin.* 3(1), 161-165. doi: http://dx.doi.org/10.5681/apb.2013.027.

[101]   Foster M, Chu A, Petocz P, Samman S. (2013 Aug 15). Effect of vegetarian diets on zinc status: a systematic review and meta-analysis of studies in humans. *Journal of the Science of Food and Agriculture.* 93(10):2362-71.

[102]   Omega-3 Fatty Acids: Fact Sheet for Health Professionals. National Institutes of Health. Last updated: October 17, 2019 https:// ods.od.nih.gov/factsheets/Omega3FattyAcids-HealthProfessional/

[103]   A. Chaddha, K. Eagle (2015 Dec) Omega-3 Fatty Acids and Heart Health. *Circulation.*

[104]   D. Siscovick, T. Raghunathan, Irena King, et al., (1995 Nov 1). Dietary Intake and Cell Membrane Levels of Long-Chain n-3 Polyunsaturated Fatty Acids and the Risk of Primary Cardiac Arrest. *JAMA.* doi: 10.1001/jama.1995.03530170043030

[105]   C. Albert, H. Campos, M. Stampfer, et al. (2002 Apr 11). Blood Levels of Long-Chain n–3 Fatty Acids and the Risk of Sudden Death. *N Engl J Med.* doi: 10.1056/NEJMoa012918

[106]   A. Erkkilä, S. Lehto, K. Pyörälä, et al. (2003 July 01) n–3 Fatty acids and 5-y risks of death and cardiovascular disease events in patients with coronary artery disease. *The American Journal of Clinical Nutrition.* doi: 10.1093/ajcn/78.1.65

[107]   Jennifer S. Lee, Po-Yin Chang, Ying Zhang, et.al. (2017 Apr). Triglyceride and HDL-C Dyslipidemia and Risks of Coronary Heart Disease and Ischemic Stroke by Glycemic Dysregulation Status: The Strong Heart Study. American Diabetes Association. doi: https://doi. org/10.2337/dc16-1958

[108]   S. Gidding, N. Allen (2019 May 29). Cholesterol and Atherosclerotic Cardiovascular Disease: A Lifelong Problem. *Journal of the American Heart Association.* doi: 10.1161/JAHA.119.012924

[109]   von Schacky, C. (2003 Mar.) The role of omega-3 fatty acids in cardiovascular disease. *Curr Atheroscler Rep 5, 139–145.* https://doi. org/10.1007/s11883-003-0086-y

[110]   Shearer G.C., Savinova O.V., Harris W. S. (2011 May): Fish oil — How does it reduce plasma triglycerides? Biochimica et Biophysica Acta (BBA) - Molecular and Cell Biology of Lipids. Volume 1821, Issue 5, May 2012, Pages 843-851. https://doi.org/10.1016/j.bbalip.2011.10.011

[111]   Back M. Omega-3 fatty acids in atherosclerosis and coronary artery disease. Future Sci. OA. 2017;3:FSO236. doi: 10.4155/fsoa-2017-0067.

[112]   F. Thies, J Garry, P. Yaqoob, et al,. (2003 Feb). Association of n-3 polyunsaturated fatty acids with stability of atherosclerotic plaques: a randomised controlled trial. Lancet. doi: 10.1016/S0140-6736(03)12468-3

[113]   G. Tackling; M. B. Borhade. (2019 May). Hypertensive Heart Disease. StatPearls.

[114]   DiNicolantonio JJ, OKeefe JImportance of maintaining a low omega-6/omega-3 ratio for reducing platelet aggregation, coagulation and thrombosisOpen Heart 2019;6:e001011. doi: 10.1136/openhrt-2019-001011

[115]   S. Sierra, F. Lara-Villoslada, M. Comalada. et al,. (2008 Mar). Dietary eicosapentaenoic acid and docosahexaenoic acid equally incorporate as decosahexaenoic acid but differ in inflammatory effects. Nutrition. doi: 10.1016/j.nut.2007.11.005

[116]   Susan K Raatz, J Bruce Redmon, et al. (2009 Jun). Enhanced absorption of omega-3 fatty acids from emulsified compared with encapsulated fish oil. J Am Diet Assoc. doi: 10.1016/j.jada.2009.03.006

[117]   Garaiova I, Guschina IA, et al. (2007 Jan.). A randomised cross-over trial in healthy adults indicating improved absorption of omega-3 fatty acids by pre-emulsification. Nutr J. doi: 10.1186/1475-2891-6-4

[118]   Institute of Medicine. (2001) Dietary Reference Intakes for Vitamin A, Vitamin K, Arsenic, Boron, Chromium, Copper, Iodine, Iron, Manganese, Molybdenum, Nickel, Silicon, Vanadium, and Zinc. Washington, DC: The National Academies Press. https://doi.org/10.17226/10026.

[119]   Warner A., Rahman A., Solsjö P. et al. (2013 October) Inappropriate heat dissipation ignites brown fat thermogenesis in mice with a mutant thyroid hormone receptor ⊠1. Proceedings of the National Academy of Sciences of the United States of America. PNAS October 1, 2013 110 (40) 16241-16246. https://doi.org/10.1073/pnas.1310300110

[120]   Krajcovicová-Kudláčková M, Bucková K, Klimes I, et al (2003 Sep). Iodine Deficiency in Vegetarians and Vegans. *Nutrition & Metabolism*. (47):183–185.

[121]   Delange F1, Bürgi H, Chen ZP, et al. (2002 Oct). World status of monitoring iodine deficiency disorders control programs. *Thyroid*. 12(10):915-24.

[122]   "FAQs about Iodine Nutrition." Accessed September 3, 2014, http://www.iccidd.org/p142000264.html.

[123]   "Iodine Deficiency," published June 4, 2012, http://www.thyroid.org/iodine-deficiency/.

[124]   "ATA Statement on the Potential Risks of Excess Iodine Ingestion and Exposure," June 5, 2013, http://www.thyroid.org/ata-statement-on-the-potential-risks-of-excess-iodine-ingestion-and-exposure/.

[125]   "Hashimoto's disease fact sheet," last updated July 16, 2012, http://womenshealth.gov/publications/our-publications/fact-sheet/hashimoto-disease.html.

[126]   Patel RB, Tannenbaum S, Viana-Tejedor A, Guo J, Im K, Morrow DA, et al. (2016 Sep 22). Serum potassium levels, cardiac arrhythmias, and mortality following non-ST-elevation myocardial infarction or unstable angina: insights from MERLIN-TIMI 36. European Heart Journal: Acute Cardiovascular Care. doi: 10.1177/2048872615624241.

[127]   Aburto NJ1, Hanson S, Gutierrez H, et al. (2013 Apr 3). Effect of increased potassium intake on cardiovascular risk factors and disease: systematic review and meta-analyses. BMJ. doi: 10.1136/bmj.f1378.

[128]   Sun Y, Byon CH, Yang Y, Bradley WE, Dell'Italia LJ, et al. (2017 Oct). Dietary potassium regulates vascular calcification and arterial stiffness. JCI Insight. doi: 10.1172/jci.insight.94920.

[129]   D'Elia L1, Barba G, Cappuccio FP, et al. (2011 Mar 8). Potassium intake, stroke, and cardiovascular disease a meta-analysis of prospective studies. J Am Coll Cardiol. doi: 10.1016/j.jacc.2010.09.070.

[130]   Rude RK. Magnesium. In: Coates PM, Betz JM, Blackman MR, et al. (2010). Encyclopedia of Dietary Supplements. 2nd ed. London and New York: Informa Healthcare.

[131]   Huang CL, Kuo E. (2007 Oct). Mechanism of hypokalemia in magnesium deficiency. J Am Soc Nephrol. doi: 10.1681/ASN.2007070792

[132]   Elena Torreggiani, Annamaria Massa, Gemma Di Pompo1 et al. (2016) Bone Abstracts - The effect of potassium citrate on human primary osteoclasts in vitro 5 P202 | doi: 10.1530/boneabs.5.P202.

[133]   Megan Ware RDN LD. (2018, January 10). "Everything you need to know about potassium." Medical News Today. Retrieved from https://www.medicalnewstoday.com/articles/287212.php.

[134]   Rude RK, Shils ME., Shike M, et al. (2006) Modern Nutrition in Health and Disease. 10th ed. *Lippincott Williams & Wilkins*, 2006:223-247.

[135]   Yu Zheng, Hong Zhou, James R.K. Modzelewski, et al. (2007 Oct) Accelerated Bone Resorption, Due to Dietary Calcium Deficiency, Promotes Breast Cancer Tumor Growth in Bone. American Association for Cancer Research (AACR).

[136]   Salynn Boyles, Reviewed by Louise Chang, MD (2008 September 03) Calcium Levels Predict Prostate Cancer. https://www. webmd.com/prostate-cancer/news/20080903/calcium-levels-predict-prostate-cancer#1.

[137]   "Magnesium and Heart Disease," accessed August 27, 2014, http://www.exatest.com/.

[138]   "What Is a Coronary Calcium Scan?" accessed July 18, 2014, http://www.nhlbi.nih.gov/health/health-topics/topics/cscan/.

[139]   WebMD Medical Reference Reviewed by James Beckerman, MD, FACC on July 6, 2018 What Is a Coronary Calcium Scan?

[140]   Harris Ripps, Wen Shen, (2012): *"Review: Taurine: A "very essential" amino acid."* https://www.ncbi.nlm.nih.gov/pmc/articles/ PMC3501277/

[141]   Michael A Moloney, Rowan G Casey, David H O'Donnell et al., (2010): *Two weeks taurine supplementation reverses endothelial dysfunction in young male type 1 diabetics.* AHA Journals. doi: 10.1177/1479164110375971

[142]   Shigeru Murakami, (2014). *Taurine and atherosclerosis.* https:// link.springer.com/article/10.1007%2Fs00726-012-1432-6

[143]   Mehdi Ahmadian, Valiollah Dabidi Roshan, Eadeh Ashourpore, (2017). *Taurine Supplementation Improves Functional Capacity, Myocardial Oxygen Consumption, and Electrical Activity in Heart Failure.* doi: abs/10 .1080/19390211.2016.1267059?journalCode=ijds20

[144]   Chazov EI, Malchikova LS, Lipina NV et al., (1974). *Taurine and electrical activity of the heart.* AHA Journals. doi/pdf/10.1161/res.35.3_supplement.iii-11

[145]   Wheeless' Textbook of Orthopaedics. Bone Remodeling (Last Updated 2011 Sep). http://www.wheelessonline.com/ortho/bone_remodeling.

[146]   Choi SY1, Kim D, Kang JH, Park MJ, et al. (2008 Mar). Nonalcoholic fatty liver disease as a risk factor of cardiovascular disease: relation of non-alcoholic fatty liver disease to carotid atherosclerosis. Korean J Hepatol. doi: 10.3350/kjhep.2008.14.1.77.

[147]   Wójcik-Cichy K., Koślińska-Berkan E., Piekarska A. (2018 Jan 20) The influence of NAFLD on the risk of atherosclerosis and cardiovascular diseases. Clinical and Experimental Hepatology. doi: 10.5114/ceh.2018.73155.

[148]   Patel SS, Beer S, Kearney DL, et al. (2013 Aug 21). Green tea extract: a potential cause of acute liver failure. World J Gastroenterol. doi: 10.3748/wjg.v19.i31.5174.

[149]   Green Tea. Last updated Nov 20, 2020. *Clinical and Research Information on Drug-Induced Liver Injury.* LiverTox: https://www.ncbi.nlm.nih.gov/books/NBK547925/

[150]   Navarro VJ, Barnhart H, Bonkovsky HL, et al. (2014) Liver injury from herbals and dietary supplements in the U.S. drug-induced liver injury network. Hepatology doi: 10.1002/hep.27317.

[151]   CDC Obesity Trends Among U.S. Adults Between 1985 and 2010 http://www.cdc.gov/obesity/downloads/obesity_trends_2010.ppt

[152]   https://www.niddk.nih.gov/health-information/health-statistics/overweight-obesity

[153]   Centers for Disease Control and Prevention. Overweight and Obesity. https://www.cdc.gov/obesity/index.html External link. Accessed July 25, 2017.

[154]   Flegal KM, Kruszon-Moran D, Carroll MD, Fryar CD, Ogden CL. Trends in obesity among adults in the United States, 2005 to 2014. The Journal of the American Medical Association. 2016;315(21):2284–2291. Available at http://jama.jamanetwork.com/article.aspx?articleid=2526639 External link or https://www.ncbi.nlm.nih.gov/pubmed/27272580

[155]   Ogden C, Carroll MD, Lawman, HG, Fryar CD, Kruszon-Moran D, et al. Trends in obesity among children and adolescents in the United States, 1988- 1994 through 2013- 2014. The Journal of the American Medical Association. 2016;315(21):2292–2299. Available at http://jamanetwork.com/journals/jama/fullarticle/2526638 External link or https://www.ncbi.nlm.nih.gov/pubmed/27272581

[156]   Fryar CD, Carroll MD, Ogden CL. Prevalence of overweight, obesity, and extreme obesity among adults aged 20 and over: United States, 1960–1962 through 2011–2014. National Center for Health Statistics Data, Health E-Stats, July 2016. Available at https://www.cdc.gov/nchs/data/hestat/obesity_adult_13_14/obesity_adult_13_14.htm External link. Accessed July 25, 2017.

[157]   CDC Behavioral Risk Factor Surveillance System (BRSS).

[158]   Yichao Huang, Fengjiang Sun, Hongli Tan, et al. (2019 Nov). DEHP and DINP Induce Tissue- and Gender-Specific Disturbances in Fatty Acid and Lipidomic Profiles in Neonatal Mice: A Comparative Study. Environ Sci Technol. doi: 10.1021/acs.est.9b04369

[159]   Marcia Wade. Last reviewed Aug 2016. *What Are Phthalates?* WebMD. https://www.webmd.com/a-to-z-guides/features/what-are-phthalates

[160]   Jeukendrup AE. (2010 Jul). Carbohydrate and exercise performance: the role of multiple transportable carbohydrates. *Current Opinion in Clinical Nutrition and Metabolic Care.* 13(4):452-7. doi: 10.1097/MCO.0b013e328339de9f.

[161]   Mowe M, Bohmer T, Kindt E. (1994) Reduced nutritional status in an elderly population (.70 year) is probable before disease and possibly contributes to the development of disease. *American Journal of Clinical Nutrition*

[162]   Larsson J, Unosson M, Ek A-C, Nilsson L, et al. Effect of dietary supplement on nutritional status and clinical outcome in 501 geriatric patients—a randomised study. *Clinical Nutrition* 1990; 9: 179–84.

[163]   "Multivitamin/mineral Supplements Fact Sheet for Health Professionals," last updated October 17, 2019, http://ods.od.nih.gov/factsheets/MVMS-HealthProfessional/.

[164]   Guallar E, Stranges S, Mulrow C, et al. (2013 Dec 17) Enough Is Enough: Stop Wasting Money on Vitamin and Mineral Supplements. *Annals of Internal Medicine.* 159(12):850-851. doi:10.7326/0003-4819-159-12-201312170-00011.

[165]   "A daily multivitamin is a great nutrition insurance policy," accessed July 27, 2014, http://www.hsph.harvard.edu/nutritionsource/what-should-you-eat/vitamins/.

[166]   Huang HY, Caballero B, Chang S, et al. (2006 May) The Efficacy and Safety of Multivitamin and Mineral Supplement Use to Prevent Cancer and Chronic Disease in Adults: A Systematic Review for a NIH State-of-the-Science Conference. *Annals of Internal Medicine*, 145:372-385.

[167]   Criteria used to compare multivitamin brands can be found at: http://www.multivitaminguide.org/study-methodology.html.

[168]   "Supplement," accessed Jul 25, 2014, http://www.merriam-webster.com/dictionary/supplement

[169]   Murray CW, Egan SK, Kim H, et al. (2008 Nov) US Food and Drug Administration's Total Diet Study: dietary intake of perchlorate and iodine. *J Expo Sci Environ Epidemiol.* 18(6):571-580. doi: 10.1038/sj.jes.7500648.

[170]   David A. Calhoun, Susan M. Harding. (2010 Aug). Sleep and Hypertension. Chest. doi: 10.1378/chest.09-2954

[171]   Ohkubo T, Hozawa A, Nagai K, et al. (2000 Jul.) Prediction of stroke by ambulatory blood pressure monitoring versus screening blood pressure measurements in a general population: the Ohasama study. Journal of Hypertension. doi : 10.1097/00004872-200018070-00005

[172]   Ben-Dov IZ, Kark JD, Ben-Ishay D, et al. (2007 Jun). Predictors of all-cause mortality in clinical ambulatory monitoring: unique aspects of blood pressure during sleep. Hypertension. doi : 10.1161/HYPERTENSIONAHA.107.087262

[173]   Francesco P Cappuccio, Daniel Cooper, Lanfranco D'Elia, et al. (2011 Jun.). Sleep duration predicts cardiovascular outcomes: a systematic review and meta-analysis of prospective studies. European Heart Journal. doi: 10.1093/eurheartj/ehr007

[174]   CDC. (2013 Jul 1). Sleep and Sleep Disorders. CDC, National Center for Chronic Disease Prevention and Health Promotion, Division of Population Health. http://www.cdc.gov/sleep/.

[175]   Pablos MI, Agapito MT, Gutierrez-Baraja R, et al (1996 Oct) Effect of calcium on melatonin secretion in chick pineal gland I. *Elsevier Science Direct.* 18;217(2-3):161-4. doi.org/10.1016/0304-3940(96)13101-3.

[176]   Caroline A. Jackson, PhD, et.al., (2018). *Psychological Distress and Risk of Myocardial Infarction and Stroke in the 45 and Up Study*. AHA Journals doi: 10.1161/CIRCOUTCOMES.117.004500

[177]   Rainer H Straub. (2014). Interaction of the endocrine system with inflammation: a function of energy and volume regulation. Arthritis Res Ther. doi: 10.1186/ar4484

[178]   J. Garcia-Leme and Sandra P. Farsky. (1993). *Hormonal control of inflammatory responses*. Department of Pharmacology, Institute of Biomedical Sciences, University of São Paulo. doi: 10.1155/S0962935193000250

[179]   The ESHRE Capri Workshop Group, (2006 Oct). Hormones and cardiovascular health in women. doi: 10.1093/humupd/dml028

[180]   M. Whipple, T. Lewis, K. Sutton-Tyrrell, et al. (2009 Aug 27). Hopelessness, depressive symptoms and carotid atherosclerosis in women: the Study of Women's Health Across the Nation (SWAN) Heart Study. Stroke. doi: 10.1161/STROKEAHA.109.554519

[181]   D. Phuong Do, J. B. Dowd, N. Ranjit, et al. (2010 Sep). Hopelessness, Depression, and Early Markers of Endothelial Dysfunction in U.S. adults. Psychosomatic Medicine. doi: 10.1097/PSY.0b013e3181e2cca5

[182]   Tips to Manage Anxiety and Stress. Retrieved October 26, 2020, from https://adaa.org/tips

[183]   R. De Vogli, T. Chandola, M. Marmot (2007 Oct 8) Negative aspects of close relationships and heart disease. Arch Intern Med. doi: 10.1001/archinte.167.18.1951

[184]   P. Mueller, MD, D. Plevak, MD, T.Rummans, MD (2001 Dec) Religious Involvement, Spirituality, and Medicine: Implications for Clinical Practice. Mayo Clinic Proceedings. doiI :https://doi.org/10.4065/76.12.1225

[185]   R. Hemmati 1 2, Z. Bidel 3, M. Nazarzadeh, et al., (2019 Aug) Religion, Spirituality and Risk of Coronary Heart Disease: A Matched Case-Control Study and Meta-Analysis. J Relig Health. doi: 10.1007/s10943-018-0722-z

[186]   Bible Gateway (accessed 3030 Oct 23) https://www.biblegateway.com/passage/?search=Proverbs+3&version=ESV

[187]   American Heart Association, (Updated 2020): *"Cardiac Medications."* Retrieved from https://www.heart.org/en/health-topics/heart-attack/treatment-of-a-heart-attack/cardiac-medications

[188]   American Society of Anesthesiologists, (Updated 2020). *Heart Surgery.* Retrieved from https://www.asahq.org/whensecondscount/preparing-for-surgery/procedures/heart-surgery/

[189]   American Heart Association, (Updated 2020). *Cardiac Procedures and Surgeries.* https://www.heart.org/en/health-topics/heart-attack/treatment-of-a-heart-attack/cardiac-procedures-and-surgeries

[190]   Hadi AH, Cornelia SC, Jassim AS (2005 September) Endothelial Dysfunction: Cardiovascular Risk Factors, Therapy, and Outcome. Vascular Health and Risk Management. 1(3): 183–198. PMID: 17319104

CPSIA information can be obtained
at www.ICGtesting.com
Printed in the USA
JSHW021414170622
27188JS00002B/64